DETECTING YOUR HIDDEN ALLERGIES

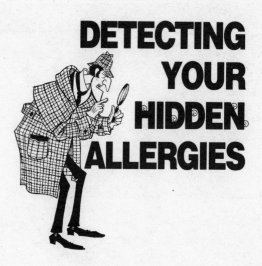

DETECTING YOUR HIDDEN ALLERGIES

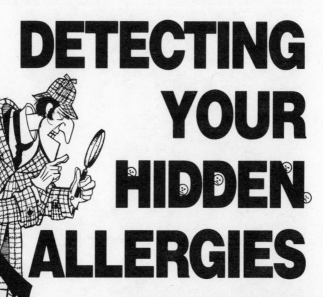

Foods you eat everyday can cause asthma, "sinus", headaches, fatigue, nervousness, digestive problems, arthritis ... and many other disorders.

By William G. Crook, M.D.

Illustrated by Cynthia Crook

Professional Books

Jackson, Tennessee 38301

Published by Professional Books, Inc., 681 Skyline Drive, Jackson, Tennessee 38301, (901) 423-5400.

ISBN: 0-933478-15-1

Manufactured in the United States of America.
1 2 3 4 5 6 7 8 9 10 — 92 91 90 89 88

Contents

About the Author

William Grant Crook, M.D. graduated from the University of Virginia School of Medicine and received his internship and residency training at the Pennsylvania Hospital in Philadelphia, Vanderbilt Hospital in Nashville, Sydenham Hospital and Johns Hopkins in Baltimore.

He has served as a Visiting Professor of Pediatrics at the Universities of California (San Francisco) and Saskatchewan and at Ohio State University. He has presented his findings relating to allergies and yeast-connected health disorders at numerous other university medical centers. These include Georgetown, U.C.L.A, Johns Hopkins, Vanderbilt and the Universities of Tennessee, Miami, Texas (San Antonio), California (San Francisco), South Alabama and South Florida.

He has also appeared at conferences of physicians and other professional and lay groups in thirty-five states and five Canadian provinces, England, Mexico, Venezuela, New Zealand, and Australia.

Doctor Crook has published over three dozen articles and reports in medical literature and has authored six books including *Answering Parents' Questions, Are You Allergic?, Can Your Child Read? Is He Hyperactive?, Tracking Down Hidden Food Allergy, The Yeast Connection—A Medical Breakthrough,* and *Solving the Puzzle of Your Hard-to-Raise Child.* A seventh book, *The Yeast Connection Cook Book,* will be published in early 1989. In addition, he has appeared on radio and television programs throughout the United States and in Canada and England.

Dr. Crook is a Diplomate of the American Board of Pediatrics, a Fellow of the American Academy of Pediatrics, the American College of Allergists and the American Academy of Environmental Medicine. He is a member of the American Academy of Allergy, the Tennessee Pediatric Society, the Tennessee Medical Association, the American Medical Association and a member of Alpha Omega Alpha. He has also served as an instructor, Department of Family Medicine, University of Tennessee, Family Practice Program, Jackson, Tennessee.

For over fourteen years (1965-1979), he wrote a nationally syndicated newspaper column, CHILD CARE (General Features and Los Angeles Times Syndicates), which appeared in cities and towns throughout the United States and Canada, including San Francisco, St. Louis, Cincinnati, Montreal, Houston, San Diego and Rochester, New York.

Doctor Crook has been referred to as a preventive medicine "crusader" who says, "The road to better health will not be found through more drugs, doctors and hospitals. Instead, it will be discovered through better nutrition and changes in life-styles."

Dr. Crook lives in Jackson, Tennessee with his wife, Betsy. They have three daughters and four grandchildren. His avocations and interests include travel, writing, golf, and bicycle riding.

Preface

In 1978, my daughter, Cynthia, and I published a 100-page, 8 x 10½ "picture book," TRACKING DOWN HIDDEN FOOD ALLERGY. Since that time this book has been used by family practitioners, pediatricians, allergists, otolaryngologists, nurses and nutritionists in evaluating and treating their patients. In addition, many people obtained a copy of TRACKING DOWN HIDDEN FOOD ALLERGY from a health food store or from a relative or friend.

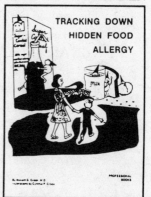

Linda B. wrote, "My son, Tom, had been bothered by a year-round stuffy nose, recurrent headaches, abdominal pain and muscle aches for years. He also was tired and irritable a good part of the time. Yet, tests and medications of several physicians hadn't helped. I'd also tried elimination diets. But organizing the diet and getting Tom to stick to it was next to impossible. Then I found TRACKING DOWN HIDDEN FOOD ALLERGY. That delightful book did everything but go out and buy foods and put them on the table."

Cynthia and I wrote TRACKING DOWN HIDDEN FOOD ALLERGY especially for children. Yet, I was pleased to learn that this book helped many adults identify their food sensitivities. Nevertheless, during the past several years, a number of physicians encouraged me to bring out an adult version. Here are a few of their comments:

"I really like TRACKING DOWN HIDDEN FOOD ALLERGY. Yet, I think adults would be more comfortable with a book geared toward them."

"I use your book all the time, but I find I have to apologize to my adult patients for the form in which this book is presented."

"Sometimes adults don't feel the book pertains to them because the simplified illustrations are geared toward children. I feel a separate book would be helpful."

Another physician commented, "I use TRACKING DOWN HIDDEN FOOD ALLERGY for both adults and children and my adult patients don't complain. I'll be interested in seeing your new version, but keep it simple . . . otherwise, my patients won't read it."

Based on these and other responses, Cynthia and I, with the help of other members of my staff, collaborated on this new book, DETECTING YOUR HIDDEN ALLERGIES. Here's a list of some of its features:

1. The simple picture book form has been retained.
2. With the help and consultation of Marge Jones*, author of THE ALLERGY SELF HELP COOKBOOK, and editor of the newsletter, MASTERING FOOD ALLERGIES—
   a. I modified and improved Elimination Diet A. For example, I suggest that legumes be eliminated as well as any food a person eats frequently.
   b. Elimination Diet B has also been updated and improved, and I suggest the grain alternatives (amaranth,

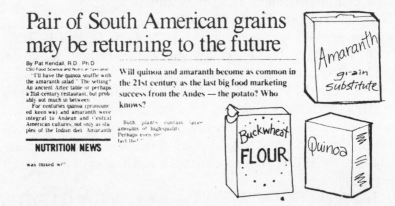

Pair of South American grains may be returning to the future

By Pat Kendall, R.D., Ph.D
CSU Food Science and Nutrition Specialist

"I'll have the quinoa soufflé with the amaranth salad." The setting? An ancient Aztec table or perhaps a 21st-century restaurant, but probably not much in between.

For centuries quinoa (pronounced keen wa) and amaranth were integral to Andean and Central American cultures, not only as staples of the Indian diet. Amaranth

NUTRITION NEWS

was mixed wi

Will quinoa and amaranth become as common in the 21st century as the last big food marketing success from the Andes — the potato? Who knows?

Both plants contain large amounts of high-quality Perhaps even m fact that

*Marge is also collaborating with me on THE YEAST CONNECTION COOKBOOK which will be published in early 1989.

buckwheat and quinoa) and the less commonly eaten vegetables (jicama, rutabaga, fennel and leeks).

   c. Meal suggestions have been modified and improved (including less fat and less frying).

   d. Extensive changes and additions were made in the recipe section.

3. I retained the question and answer section. Yet, I updated and improved it and the person asking the question is an adult with headaches, abdominal pain, muscle aches and nasal congestion, rather than a child with hyperactivity.

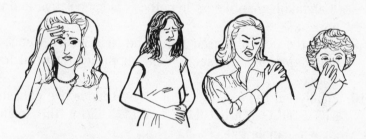

4. Cynthia and I made changes in the illustrations and the parables so that they're now adult oriented. And at the risk of being called "female chauvinists" (with the approval of a number of consultants—both male and female), we show a woman physician talking to a male patient.

5. I briefly discuss the many common food allergy masquerades including abdominal pain, muscle and joint pain, headaches, urinary problems, irritability, nervousness and fatigue.

6. I wrote a new section which contains descriptions of hidden food allergies in the medical and lay literature dating back to the Old Testament.

7. Many of today's foods are contaminated. I discuss this subject in The Chemical Problem and a new

section, More on the Chemical Contamination of Your Food and What You Can Do About It.

8. I include a discussion of the controversial candida-human illness hypothesis in a new section entitled, "Hidden Food Allergies and The Yeast Connection." Yet, I realize that many physicians (including the Practice Standards Committee of the American Academy of Allergy and Immunology) state that the "Candida-human illness hypothesis is speculative and unproven."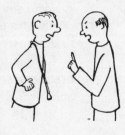

9. With the help of Marge Jones and Nell Sellers, I updated and expanded the section on shopping tips and food sources.

10. Finally—at the suggestion of many friends, we published DETECTING YOUR HIDDEN ALLERGIES in this smaller, easy-to-handle size.

This book is designed especially for adults. Yet, it retains the simple illustrations and should be equally useful in working with children. The big-page edition of TRACKING DOWN HIDDEN FOOD ALLERGY will be available for those who prefer it.

A Special Message to the Physician

When I began practicing medicine in my hometown, Jackson, Tennessee, in February, 1949, I knew absolutely nothing about hidden or delayed-onset hidden food allergies. I remained unaware of such allergies until the autumn of 1955.

At that time I was struggling (unsuccessfully) to help Mack, a 12-year-old boy who lived in my neighborhood. Mack's complaints included severe headaches, fatigue, irritability, abdominal pain and muscle aches. When a comprehensive evaluation showed no apparent cause for his symptoms, I said to his mother, "Aileen, I feel Mack has an emotional problem."

During the discussion which ensued, Aileen said, "Dr. Crook, I have a suggestion. Let's take milk out of Mack's diet. I think it could be causing his symptoms. Here's why I suspect milk. When Mack was an infant, he developed a scaly rash on his cheeks and other parts of his body. His pediatrician put him on a soy bean formula and the rash disappeared.

"When we gave Mack a cow's milk formula again, his rash returned. So we kept Mack off milk indefinitely. Mack never consumed dairy products until this fall. Then, at the suggestion of his teacher, Mack began drinking several glasses of milk a day and that's when his symptoms began.

"Another reason why I think milk might bother Mack is that milk problems run in the family. Milk gives me a headache and my mother diarrhea and my grandmother develops mucus in her throat when she drinks milk. If she keeps drinking it, she gets an attack of bronchitis."

So Aileen began to experiment with Mack's diet and to try him off and on milk. Three weeks later, she called and gave me this report, "I took milk out of Mack's diet. He felt worse for a couple of days—more headaches and fatigue. Then he gradually began to feel better and after a week, he was like a different child. No headaches, belly aches, irritability or fatigue. When he drank milk again, his symptoms returned. When he avoided milk, his symptoms went away. I'm sure that milk disagrees with him."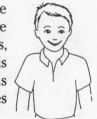

A few weeks later, I came across two articles in the November 1954 issue of the PEDIATRIC CLINICS OF NORTH AMERICA. One was a report by Susan Dees of Duke University which described nervous system disorders related to food allergy; the second was an article by Frederic Speer of the University of Kansas entitled, *The Allergic Tension-Fatigue Syndrome.*

Dees described a variety of nervous system disorders (including convulsions) which in some patients had been found to be food related. Speer told of patients with headache, fatigue, muscle aches, irritability, abdominal pain and other systemic nervous system symptoms who improved when they avoided foods they were eating every day.

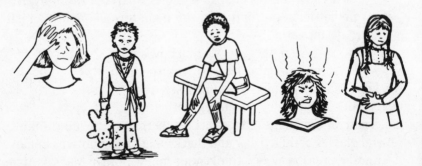

Speer reviewed the medical literature and listed 21 references at the end of his article. I was fascinated. So I drove to Memphis to the medical library of the University of Tennessee and looked up most of the articles Speer had cited. And like Speer, the authors of these reports told of food-related, systemic and nervous system symptoms.

So I began to search for patients in my practice with similar problems and I was amazed to find many of them. I reported my findings on 23 food-sensitive youngsters at the Allergy Section Meeting of the American Academy of Pediatrics in Chicago in 1958.

I subsequently published a paper based on a study of 50 such children in PEDIATRICS in 1961. Included was a scientific study on Mack, my first patient. During the past 25 years, my interest in hidden food allergies continued and I published my observations in both the medical and lay literature.

During this time, most physicians paid little attention to the relationship of hidden food allergies to headache, abdominal pain, muscle aches and other systemic and nervous system symptoms. Yet, during the past five to ten years, hidden food allergies and the importance of elimination diets in identifying them have "come into the medical mainstream." (See page 195.)

I freely admit that tracking down hidden food allergies won't solve all of the complaints of your difficult patients. Yet, I think you'll be amazed and gratified—just as I was—when you see how many of them respond to carefully designed and properly executed elimination diets.*

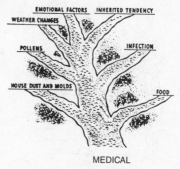

MEDICAL
MAINSTREAM

---

*See also: Descriptions of Hidden Food Allergies in the Medical and Lay Literature (page 161), Food Allergies and Food Hypersensitivities, Elimination Diets Come Into the Medical Mainstream (page 195), Hidden Food Allergies and The Yeast Connection (page 200) and the Medical References (page 213).

What This Book Is All About

If you (or your child) are bothered by fatigue, headache, drowsiness, depression, irritability, inability to concentrate, hyperactivity (or other nervous system symptoms), dark circles under your eyes, nasal congestion, frequent or recurrent ear infections or bronchitis, pallor (in the absence of anemia), wheezing, coughing, recurring abdominal pain, muscle aching, and/or urinary symptoms, go to your doctor for a careful check-up, including a history and physical examination, complete blood count, urinalysis and tuberculin test. Your physician may also feel that a chest x-ray, thyroid tests and other blood studies are necessary.

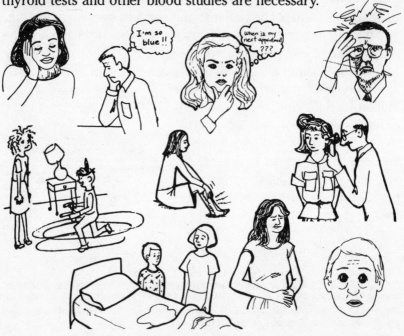

But before undergoing more complex, expensive and painful tests or procedures, including gastrointestinal x-rays, urinary tract x-rays, electroencephalographic examinations and brain scans, psychiatric evaluation or surgery, try an elimination diet and see if your symptoms get better.

Also try an elimination diet before you settle for symptomatic relief with tranquilizers, mood elevators or other drugs which may help some of your symptoms without getting at their cause.

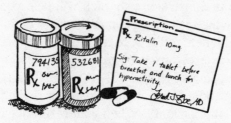

This book is written especially for adults, although you can certainly use it in working with your child. It provides you with specific instructions for carrying out elimination diets. *By following instructions in this book, you can usually determine whether or not your symptoms are caused by adverse or allergic reactions to foods you're eating every day.*

On pages 50–57, you'll find pictures and food lists which will help you know what foods you can and cannot eat on Elimination Diet A—a diet which avoids foods which commonly cause hidden allergies in Americans (milk, corn, wheat, egg, yeast, citrus, legumes, beet and cane sugar, coffee and tea); Diet A also avoids food dyes, flavors, additives and alcoholic beverages.

On pages 71-72, you'll find shopping tips which tell you where to obtain the foods you need for Elimination Diet A (on page 91 you'll find further shopping tips).

On pages 74–77 and pages 82–89, you'll find food lists, illustrations and menus for Elimination Diet B (sometimes called the Rare Food or "Cave Man" Diet). **In carrying out**

this diet, avoid any and every food you eat more than once a week.

On pages 90 and 91–95, you'll find a list of food sources which will help you or your food store obtain foods you'll need for your diet.

On pages 96–112, you'll find questions and answers which will help you prepare menus and obtain the cooperation of other family members.

You'll also find instructions which will help you keep accurate records and which tell you when and how to eliminate foods from your diet and when and how to add them back so as to find out if your symptoms are caused by foods you're eating.

On pages 115 and 121–126, you'll find the story or parable about Maria which illustrates the important concept of "allergic load." When your resistance is high and your load of allergy troublemakers is low, you're apt to remain symptom free and well. Yet, when your allergy troublemakers combine, they overcome your resistance and make you sick.

On pages 116–120, the parable, Tom's Cow's Milk Allergy, illustrates another important allergy principle which applies especially to hidden food allergy. Fortunately, even though you're allergic to a common food (such as milk, corn or wheat) if you avoid the food for several months, your sensitivity to the food decreases (like a fire that dies down). So most allergy sufferers regain tolerance to a food they're allergic to if they avoid it for several months and then eat it in smaller amounts every 4 to 7 days.

On pages 134–135, you'll find information about rotated diets including examples of such diets.

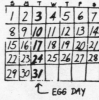

S	M	T	W	T	F	S
1	2	3	4	5	6	7
8	9	10	11	12	13	14
15	16	17	18	19	20	21
22	23	24	25	26	27	28
29	30	31				

⌐ EGG DAY

To detect your hidden food allergies, you must keep a symptom diary.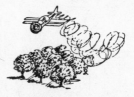

a. Begin your diary at least 3 days before you start eliminating foods.
b. Maintain your diary while you're eliminating foods.
c. Continue it while you're returning foods to your diet.

You'll find suggestions which may help you stick to your diet. These suggestions involve a program of behavior modification which will make you less apt to cheat.

Many of today's foods are chemically contaminated. I discuss this subject in the Chemical Problem and a new section, More on the Chemical Contamination of Your Food and What You Can Do About It. (See pages 138–146.)

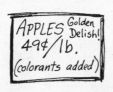

Three new sections have been added to this book:

1. Descriptions of Hidden Food Allergies in the Medical and Lay Literature.
2. Food Allergies, Food Hypersensitivities and Elimination Diets Come into the Medical Mainstream.
3. Hidden Food Allergies and The Yeast Connection.

Although these sections were designed especially for physicians and other professionals, they'll interest you and everyone working to identify and manage their hidden allergies.

What Is Allergy?

The term "allergy" was coined in 1906 by Austrian pediatrician Clemens von Pirquet who put together two Greek words, *allos* (other) and *ergon* (work or action). *So an allergic person reacts to substances that don't bother other people.*

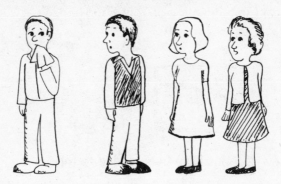

When you or your child develop an allergy to a substance—such as ragweed, ragweed is called an allergen. Substances of a different sort in your body which react with allergens are called antibodies.

When *allergens* and *antibodies* come together, reactions which occur resemble "tiny explosions." Histamine and other chemicals are released throughout the body. These chemicals (often called "mediators") make automatic muscles tighten up and go into spasm. And they cause blood vessels to leak fluid, and glands in the nose, bronchial tubes and other parts of the body to put out excessive mucus.

WHEN . . .

Allergens 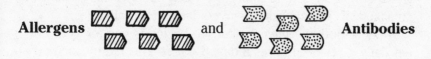 **and** **Antibodies**

come together

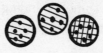

they produce
Histamine and other substances

which are released and act on . . .

Blood Vessels   *Circular Muscles*   *Mucous Glands*

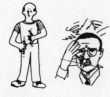

causing
ALLERGIC SYMPTOMS

When you are highly sensitive to a food, such as strawberries or fish, the allergic reaction occurs rapidly . . . even violently . . . in a few seconds to a few minutes. Symptoms produced include rash, swelling, sneezing, wheezing, severe abdominal cramps, vomiting, and fainting. Such a reaction is termed an *obvious food allergy*. No elimination diets are needed to identify this sort of allergy.

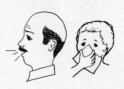

Many, many times more common are the food allergies, hyper-sensitivities and other adverse reactions described in this book.* I call them "hidden food allergies." Such allergies have also been "masked," "variable," or "delayed-onset" food allergies.

Hidden food allergies are caused by foods you (or your child) eat daily, or several times a day. If you're affected by such an allergy, you're apt to be sensitive to your favorite foods. And strange as it seems, you may be addicted to the foods which are making you sick. And like the cigarette or narcotic addict, you're apt to feel better after you eat a food you're allergic to.

Accordingly, detecting a hidden food allergy requires carefully planned and executed elimination diets. This book is designed to help you carry out such diets and to give you a clearer understanding of hidden food allergies, how to recognize them, prevent them and treat them.

---

*Four types of allergic reactions have been identified and classified. One of these (Type I) is mediated through a blood fraction called "IgE." Reactions of this type produce positive scratch tests in individuals sensitive to pollens and other inhalants, and much less commonly in individuals sensitive to food. However, *many and perhaps most individuals who show the adverse food reactions discussed in this book will not show positive scratch* or other immunologic tests.

At this time (1988), in spite of studies by many investigators during the past few years, many of the mechanisms and explanations for these food reactions remain obscure. Since they may not involve antigen and antibody reactions, many immunologists and other physicians prefer to call these food reactions "intolerances," "hypersensitivities" or "adverse reactions."

Acknowledgments

I wish to especially acknowledge the inspiration and help I received from Theron Randolph, the late Albert Rowe, Sr., the late Jerome Glaser, the late Frederic Speer and the late William C. Deamer. Each of these physicians invited me to visit them and observe their methods of caring for their allergic patients—more especially, those with hidden food allergies.

I'm also indebted to Elmer Cranton of Trout Dale, Virginia and Harold Hedges of Little Rock, Arkansas. Each of these physicians reviewed the manuscript of this book and have shared their knowledge and experiences with me on many occasions. Through their own publications and lectures, they have helped spread the word about hidden food allergies to thousands of physicians.

I also wish to acknowledge the contributions of Marge Jones, R.N., author of THE ALLERGY SELF-HELP COOKBOOK and editor of the newsletter, MASTERING FOOD ALLERGIES. Marge carefully reviewed and edited the manuscript of this book and provided me with many helpful menus and recipes.

I want to especially thank Nell Sellers who helped with research, editing, cooking and menu preparation and Charlotte Jaquet who typed and retyped the manuscript many many times. I'm also grateful for the help and encouragement of Brent Lay, Nancy Moss, Brenda Harris, Denny Spencer, Georgia Deaton and Alice Spragins.

I'm also grateful to hundreds of my patients and other friends who have shared their experiences with me and to dozens of physicians and other professionals including:

Lorraine Abbey, Leonard Baker, Sidney Baker, Dean Baldwin, Iris Bell, Robert Boxer, Cecil Bradley, J. C. Breneman, James Brodsky, Jonathan Brostoff, Dor Brown, Robert Buckley, J. D. Bullock, Harold Buttram, Mary Callahan, M. B. Campbell, Jeremiah Chunn, Irene Colquhoun, Pat Connolly, Stephen Davies, Belinda Dawes, Susan Dees, the late Lawrence Dickey, Robert Dockhorn, Paul Dragul, Bruce Duncan, the late Ben Feingold, Hobart Feldman, Ronald Finn, Trish Frederick, O. L. Frick, Leo Galland, Zane Gard, John Gerrard, Tom Glasgow, Natalie Golos, Ellen Grant, Howard Hagglund, Clyde Hawley, Douglas Heiner, John Henderson, Amelia Nathan Hill, Jesse M. Hilsen, Abram Hoffer, Patricia Holabough, Harris Hosen, Beatrice Trum Hunter, Martha Hutson, W. Kaufman, William T. Kniker, George Kroker, Barry Kronman, Alan Levin, Allan Lieberman, the late Steven Lockey, Richard Mabray, Richard Mackarness, Marshall Mandell, John Mansfield, Tatsuo Matsumura, L. M. McEwen, Charles McGee, John McGovern, Joseph McGovern, I. C. Menzies, John Michael, Joseph Miller, Maureen Minchen, David Morris, Jean Monro, Nick Nonas, Gary Oberg, John O'Brian, James O'Shea, Frank Oski, W. H. Philpott, S. Pilar, Doris Rapp, William Rea, Chris Redding, Eli Revai, Joyce Riley, C. Rippere, Sherry Rogers, Michael Rosenberg, Alexander Roth, Albert Rowe, Jr., Phyllis Saifer, Douglas Sandberg, Sam Sanders, Jennifer Scott, George Shambaugh, Sara Sloan, Laura Stevens, J. Allen Stewart, Del Stigler, Robert Stroud, Garland Stroup, Morton Teich, Ann Tenenbaum, Steven Tobler, Olive Tompson, John Toth, Donald Toures, John Parks Tworbridge, C. Orian Truss, Louis Tuft, Walter Tunnesen, Jr., Francis Waickman, Walter Ward, James Willoughby, Aubrey Worrell, Jonathan Wright, Ray Wunderlich, Alfred Zamm.

Dedication

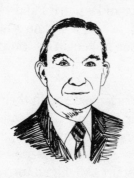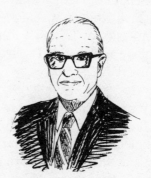

This book is dedicated to two food allergy pioneers who served as my mentors:

The late William C. Deamer, M.D., Professor of Pediatrics, University of California, San Francisco.

The late Frederic C. Speer, M.D., Clinical Professor of Pediatrics, University of Kansas and University of Missouri, Kansas City.

I would also like to recognize and pay special tribute to fourteen other physicians including six from academic medicine and eight from practice.

Academicians. During the past one to two decades, these physicians have played an important role in bringing hidden or delayed-onset food allergies and/or hypersensitivities into the medical mainstream:

Sami L. Bahna, M.D., Chairman of the Food Allergy Committee of the American College of Allergists, Chairman, Department of Allergy and Immunology, The Cleveland Clinic Foundation, Cleveland, Ohio.

Oscar Lee Frick, M.D., Professor of Pediatrics, University of California, San Francisco.

John W. Gerrard, M.D., Emeritus Professor of Pediatrics, University of Saskatchewan.

Douglas Heiner, M.D., Professor of Pediatrics, University of California School of Medicine (Los Angeles).

William T. Kniker, M.D., Professor of Pediatrics and Microbiology, University of Texas Health Science Center, San Antonio.

Douglas Sandberg, M.D., Professor of Pediatrics, University of Miami.

Allergy practitioners. These physicians, through their lectures and publications and through their influence and leadership in various medical organizations, have helped physicians, other professionals and the public learn more about hidden food allergies:

James C. Breneman, M.D., Galesburg, Michigan, private practice. Dr. Breneman served as Chairman of the Food Allergy Committee of the American College of Allergists for many years and continues to serve on this important committee.

Elmer Cranton, M.D., Trout Dale, Virginia, private practice. Editor, Journal of Advancement in Medicine.

Robert Dockhorn, M.D., Kansas City, Kansas, private practice. Past President of the American College of Allergists.

Harold Hedges, M.D., Little Rock, Arkansas, private practice.

James C. Kemp, M.D., San Diego, California, private practice. Clinical Professor of Allergy, University of California.

Doris Rapp, M.D., Buffalo, New York, private practice. Researcher, author and lecturer. Clinical Associate Professor of Pediatrics, State University of New York at Buffalo.

George E. Shambaugh, Jr., M.D. Hinsdale, Illinois, private practice, Professor of Otolaryngology (Emeritus), Northwestern University, Past President, American Academy of Otolaryngic Allergy.

Robert M. Stroud, M.D., Daytona Beach, Florida, private practice. Clinical Professor of Medicine, University of Florida (Gainesville).

A Special Message To Readers

Elimination diets were first described by Daniel in the Old Testament. Countless people since that time have found that what they eat (or do not eat) affects the way they feel.

I've helped thousands of my patients during the past thirty years using the elimination diets described in this book. And I have never encountered a serious or dangerous reaction—even though the diets were carried out by my patients at home.

So you can carry out an elimination diet with safety and confidence. Moreover, carrying out such a diet is safer than getting into your car and driving to your shopping center—or to your physician's office.

BUT IF—

1. you've ever had asthma (especially if it has been severe)
2. you've ever had hives or swelling (especially involving lips, tongue or throat)
3. you've ever been troubled by severe skin rashes of any type
4. you're troubled by heart disease or a serious health problem of any type—

consult your physician and get his help and cooperation before carrying out the diets described in this book.

Elimination diets and challenges in infants, especially those under one year of age, or in individuals with anorexia, bulimia, or other severe, chronic health disorders should not be attempted without help, consultation and supervision by a physician.

Reports on food allergies and hypersensitivities have appeared in the medical and lay literature during the past 70 years. Dozens of these reports are listed in the Reference section pages 213–220.

Suggestions for further reading on food allergies can be found in the Reading List located on pages 210–212.

Hidden Food Allergies Can Make You Sick

Common Manifestations of Hidden Food Allergies

Allergic reactions resemble an iceberg. About $1/7$ of the iceberg is visible above the water while the remaining part is submerged.

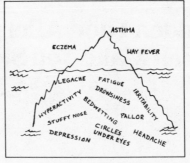

THE ALLERGY ICEBERG

Obvious allergies, including asthma, hayfever, eczema and urticaria (hives) resemble the part of the iceberg above the water. Respiratory allergies are easy to recognize when you sneeze, cough, itch, break out in a rash or wheeze when you play with the cat, cut the grass, go on a picnic in ragweed season or rummage around in the attic. And you can identify your obvious food allergies if you swell, itch and break out in hives when you eat lobster, strawberries or cashew nuts.

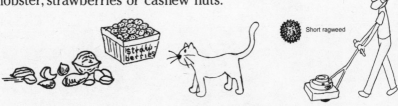

Short ragweed

By contrast, hidden food allergies, like the parts of the iceberg under the surface of the water, won't be found unless you search for them. And to succeed in your search, you'll need to carry out a carefully-designed elimination diet.

If your symptoms get better when you avoid some of your favorite foods and return when you eat them again, you'll understand many of your puzzling problems.

Here are a few of the common manifestations of hidden food allergies:

Pallor and Allergic "Shiners"

People with anemia look pale. So do people with kidney disease, malnutrition and other chronic health disorders, even when they aren't anemic.

Hidden food allergies can make you look that way too. Here's why: Clear fluid leaks from your capillaries, giving your face a pale, puffy and pasty appearance.

So if you look pale (especially if you have dark shadows or bags under your eyes and a stuffy nose) hidden food allergies may be responsible for your pallor. When these allergies are brought under control, your color will usually improve.

Abdominal Pain

Many different things can make your stomach ache. And if your pain persists and you go to your physician for a checkup, he may suspect a stomach ulcer, gall stones, parasites in your intestines, a hidden kidney disorder, Crohn's disease, constipation, at times alternating with loose stools (so called functional bowel syndrome), rectal itching (perianal), or excessive gas. Yet, when your x-rays and other studies are "normal," some physicians tend to blame abdominal pain on "nerves" or a spastic colon.

Although emotional stress can cause digestive symptoms, a number of physicians have pointed out that recurrent abdominal pain is often caused by food allergies and other adverse food reactions.

In a recent report from England, Virginia Alun Jones and J. O. Hunter, in summarizing their studies of irritable bowel syndrome and Crohn's disease, commented,

"Objective food intolerances have been shown by a number of independent workers to occur in some patients with irritable bowel syndrome. *The trial of an exclusion diet should be considered in all patients with unexplained colonic pain or diarrhea.*"

You should especially suspect a hidden food allergy if your recurrent abdominal pain is accompanied by nasal congestion, pallor, dark circles under your eyes, fatigue, headaches and muscle aches.

Allergic abdominal pain is apparently caused by tightening of the smooth (circular) muscles which surround every part of your digestive tract. Other mechanisms may also be involved including increased mucous gland secretion and leakage of fluid from small capillaries.

So before blaming your abdominal pain on an emotional cause, rule out hidden food allergies. Usually such allergies are caused by milk or other foods you're eating every day.

Muscle and Joint Pains

Many disorders can cause aching or swelling in the muscles or joints. These include orthopedic abnormalities, rheumatoid arthritis, osteoarthritis, inadequate exercise or too much exercise without proper preconditioning. However, hidden food allergies are a common and often overlooked cause of musculoskeletal discomfort, and can cause increase of symptoms in any type of arthritis.

Over fifty years ago, the late Albert H. Rowe, Sr., M.D., of Oakland, California first described aching muscles, bones and joints caused by food allergy. Since that time many physicians have noted that allergies, especially hidden food allergies, often cause painful muscles and joints. Joseph Bullock, M.D., William Deamer, M.D., O. L. Frick, M.D. and associates of the University of

California, San Francisco, also described musculoskeletal discomfort caused by hidden food allergies. They commented,

"We've seen patients who have been diagnosed as rheumatic because of leg aches and fever. One patient had a muscle biopsy because of leg ache and fatigability . . . (His) symptoms disappeared following the eliminiation of chocolate and milk from the diet."

More recently, Kroker, Stroud, Panush and Hill have noted that musculoskeletal symptoms (even arthritis) could be related to adverse food reactions.

How can food allergies cause musculoskeletal symptoms? Here are possible explanations: The blood vessels that supply oxygen and other nutrients to the muscle and joint tissues are surrounded by the same circular muscles that surrounded the bronchial tubes, intestines and bladder. When these muscles go in to spasm, tissues may be deprived of oxygen and pain may occur. Pain and swelling may also develop when capillaries leak fluid into the tissues.

Persistent Colds, Bronchitis, Asthma and "Sinus"
You can suspect an allergic respiratory disorder if you're bothered by:

1. Frequent sneezing and nasal itching, chronic nasal congestion or stuffiness, often called "sinus" problems.
2. Night cough that continues for days and weeks at a time.
3. Cough on exertion.
4. Recurrent attacks of asthma or bronchitis.
5. Other family members do not seem to "catch" your cold, and minor colds hang on and on.

Respiratory allergies are commonly caused by house dust mites, animal danders, molds, pollens and other inhalants. They can also be aggravated by chemical fumes and odors including tobacco smoke and perfume. *Yet, foods you eat every day can also play an important role in causing respiratory symptoms.*

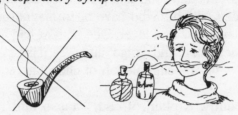

In his award-winning presentation in 1970, Bill Deamer emphasized the role of foods in causing respiratory symptoms. He noted that foods were a factor in an estimated 40% of children with asthma and *the only cause* in 10%. (See also pages 174–175.)

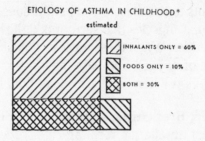

ETIOLOGY OF ASTHMA IN CHILDHOOD*
estimated

INHALANTS ONLY = 60%

FOODS ONLY = 10%

BOTH = 30%

And in presentations at the annual meetings of the American Academy of Allergists in 1986 and again in 1987, Ted Kniker noted that both chronic rhinitis and asthma in adults were often food related. (See also pages 191–194.)

Headaches

If you're bothered by recurrent headaches, you may have consulted your family physician, an eye specialist, an ear, nose and throat specialist or a neurologist. In trying to identify the cause of your headaches, studies of various sorts (including sinus x-rays, skull x-rays, brain wave tests, or CAT scans) may have been carried out.

When these studies are normal, your physician is apt to conclude that your headaches are caused by stress. Yet, studies by

*W. C. Deamer, *Pediatrics*, 48:930, 1971.

McGovern and Haywood, Monro, Egger, Carter, Wilson, Soothill, Grant and others show that headaches in both children and adults are usually related to food allergies and other adverse food reactions.

Urinary Problems

You'll probably be surprised to know that food allergies can play an important role in causing diseases and disorders in kidneys, bladder and other parts of your urinary tract. Yet, such a relationship has been described by many observers during the past fifty years. For example, Bray in England over fifty years ago noted that bedwetting in children was often related to food allergies. Subsequently, this same relationship has been noted by other observers including Breneman* and Gerrard.**

Here's what seems to happen: When a person eats a food he's allergic to, the muscular coat around the bladder contracts. This makes the bladder smaller and keeps it from holding a normal amount of urine. As a result, the child will urinate more often during the daytime and may wet the bed at night. Although adults rarely wet the bed, a similar mechanism can make you urinate more often during the daytime and get up to go to the bathroom at night.

---

*Breneman: For many years, Chairman of the Food Allergy Committee of the American College of Allergists, author of BASICS OF FOOD ALLERGY. In 1959, Breneman reported for the first time in the American medical literature on the role of foods in causing nocturnal enuresis (G.P. 20:84, 1959). See also references.

**Gerrard: Professor of Pediatrics Emeritus, University of Saskatchewan, member of the Adverse Food Committee of the American Academy of Allergy and Immunology. Author of *Understanding Allergies and Food Allergy: New Perspectives*. Gerrard first published his observations on food-related enuresis in the Canadian Medical Association Journal, Volume 101, page 269. See also references.

Allergy may also play an important part in causing other disturbances of the urinary tract including recurrent urinary tract infections.* Here's a possible mechanism. Allergic spasm of the sphincter muscle may keep you from emptying your bladder completely which may, in turn, make you more prone to urinary tract infections. Moreover, Tatsuo Matsumura, a Japanese allergist, has carried out scientific studies which show that albumin in the urine may be related to food allergies and Douglas Sandberg, of the University of Miami has described other urological problems which are related to food allergies.

Allergy can cause still other genito-urinary symptoms. The cause of such symptoms include foods and food coloring and additives.

A final note: Recently I saw a patient with extreme urinary frequency that had been diagnosed as interstitial cystitis. Following an elimination diet and challenge, her symptoms were markedly improved. Then when she added wheat and corn her symptoms flared up.

Irritability and Nervousness

Food-related nervous symptoms in both children and adults have been described by countless observers during the twentieth century. For example, Hare in Australia in 1904 told of people with many types of nervous symptoms who improved following changes in their diet. Subsequently, in the next two decades, several American physicians described nervous system allergies. How-

---

*Elmer Cranton comments: "Many patients with repeated bouts of urinary frequency, urgency and painful urination do *not* have infection. The symptoms of allergy can closely mimic cystitis, urethritis and prostatitis. Such patients are often treated with repeated courses of antibiotics because of the assumption that infection is the cause. Antibiotics cause yeast overgrowth and this, in turn, aggravates underlying allergies.

"A culture and colony count on a clean-catch, mid-stream urine specimen, within a few minutes of voiding, should show significant numbers of bacteria before antibiotics are used."

ever, few physicians were aware of such reactions until Albert Rowe, Sr., began to write about and talk about the food/mood connection in 1930.

During the past fifty years, the Rowe observations have been confirmed by Rinkel, Randolph, Speer, Deamer, Gerrard, Rapp 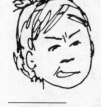 and many others. In the late 1950s, I learned for the first time that irritability, overactivity and other nervous symptoms were often food related. Here's a typical comment from the wife of one of my patients.

"If my husband, John, eats chocolate every day, by the end of the fourth day he becomes grumpy and irritable. In fact, so irritable that I can't stand to be around him. What's more, he doesn't even like himself. John also seems jittery and shaky and unable to concentrate on his work. When he stops eating chocolate, his whole personality changes.

Food induced nervous system symptoms include restlessness and an inability to sit still. Some adults may show symptoms resembling those seen in the hyperactive child.* Others with food induced nervous system problems show symptoms mainly affecting their moods. So they're irritable, argumentative and unable to be pleased.

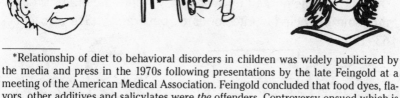

---

*Relationship of diet to behavioral disorders in children was widely publicized by the media and press in the 1970s following presentations by the late Feingold at a meeting of the American Medical Association. Feingold concluded that food dyes, flavors, other additives and salicylates were *the* offenders. Controversy ensued which is still going on today (1988).

Other observers including Crook, Rapp and Egger, like Feingold, found that food dyes frequently cause hyperactive behavior in children. Yet, they emphasize the role of sensitivity to many other foods in causing behavioral disturbances. (You'll find a full discussion of the diet/behavior relationship in SOLVING THE PUZZLE OF YOUR HARD-TO-RAISE CHILD by William G. Crook, M.D and Laura Stevens, Professional Books, Jackson, Tennessee and Random House, New York, New York, 1987.)

Food induced nervous system symptoms can make people unpleasant to have around. Because of their disagreeable personality traits, such individuals are apt to be shunned or rejected by family members, friends and associates.

Fatigue

Nervous system allergies can cause a person to be up or down. In many people, symptoms of irritability and overactivity alternate with feelings of fatigue, drowsiness, weakness, malaise, and depression. Theron Randolph described these alternating symptoms in children in 1947 and in 1954, Frederic Speer coined a term to describe them: The Allergic Tension-Fatigue Syndrome.

Allergic fatigue can make you wake up tired and remain tired all day regardless of how much sleep you get. And your fatigue may continue even though you like your job and the emotional climate at home is a good one.

If you're always tired, it's important to make sure you aren't suffering from anemia, thyroid deficiency or some other hidden illness. When such disorders are ruled out and you are bothered by headaches, muscle aches, nasal congestion, a pale color and allergic shiners, your fatigue is probably related to hidden food allergies.

After reading the reports of these food allergy pioneers in 1956, I began to look for patients with food-related fatigue in my practice. I was amazed to find that many of my tired, listless, drowsy, sluggish patients perked up when they stopped eating (or drinking) some of their favorite foods or beverages. (See also pages 163–194.)

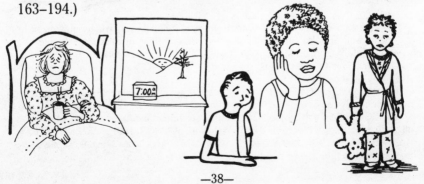

How to Find Out If Your Symptoms Are Caused by Something You're Eating

You Can Suspect A Hidden Food Allergy When You (or Your Child)...

develop dark circles or "bags" under your eyes,

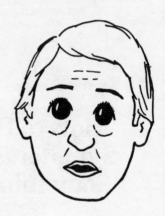

sniff, snort, clear your throat or push your nose up.

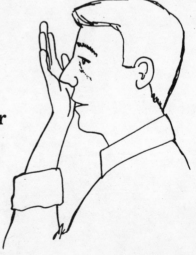

are nervous, irritable or "spaced out"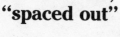

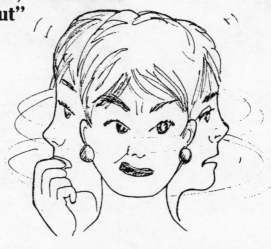

are tired, droopy, drowsy or depressed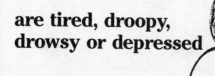

complain of headache,
stomachache or muscle
and joint pains.

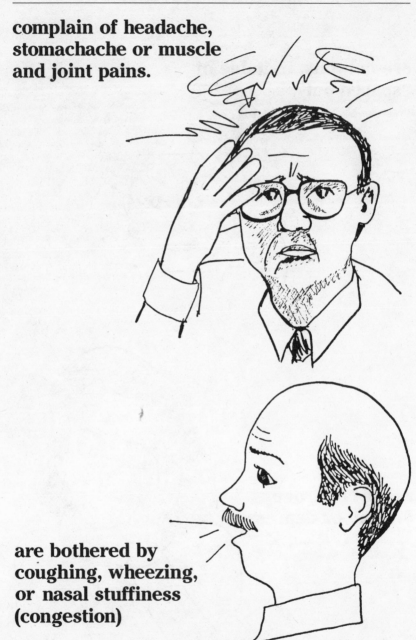

are bothered by
coughing, wheezing,
or nasal stuffiness
(congestion)

were plagued by
irritability and frequent
digestive and
respiratory problems or
ear infections in infancy
and/or early childhood
or at any time in life

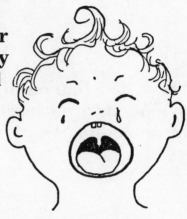

. . . or other members
of your family are
bothered by allergies

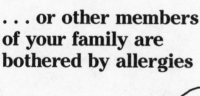

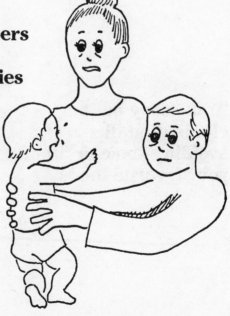

You're Probably Asking . . .

"How do I find out if my symptoms are caused by something I eat?"

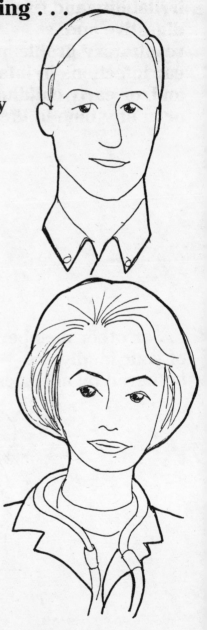

"You carry out an elimination diet avoiding some or all of your favorite foods."

**"What will I look for?
. . . How will I know I'm
allergic?"**

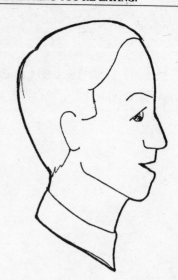

**"If you're allergic to the
foods you avoid, your
symptoms will improve
or disappear. And they
will return when you
eat the foods again."**

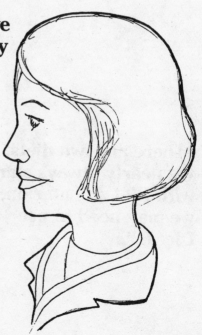

**"What foods can I eat
on the diet?"**

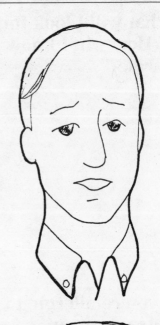

**"There are two diets.
We nearly always start
with Diet A. Later on,
we may need to use
Diet B."**

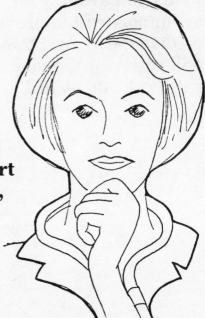

ELIMINATION DIETS

ELIMINATION DIET A

The diet instructions on the following pages provide you with pictures and lists of:

1. Foods you (or your child) can eat.
2. Foods you (or your child) must avoid.

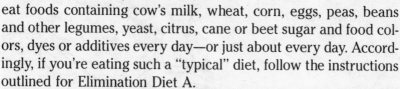

These diet instructions were designed for the "average" person who lives in the United States, Canada, the British Isles, Australia and New Zealand. And many such individuals eat foods containing cow's milk, wheat, corn, eggs, peas, beans and other legumes, yeast, citrus, cane or beet sugar and food colors, dyes or additives every day—or just about every day. Accordingly, if you're eating such a "typical" diet, follow the instructions outlined for Elimination Diet A.

But you're unique and if you eat bananas, apples, potatoes, rice, beef, lamb, chicken (or other favorite foods) every single day, you'll need to modify these instructions so that you'll be eliminating the foods which are most apt to be causing your symptoms.

Instructions for preparing foods indicated by an asterisk can be found in the recipe section (pages 148–160).

Foods you (or your child) can eat

Vegetables
(any but corn, peas, beans
and other legumes)

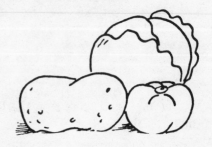

Fruits
(any but citrus)

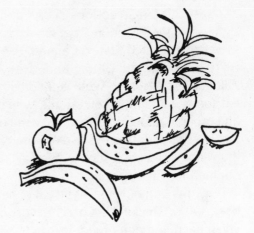

Meats
(any but bacon, sausage,
hot dogs or luncheon
meats)

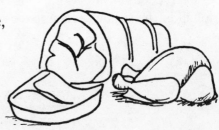

**Special Bread and
Crackers**
(containing no wheat,
rye or corn)

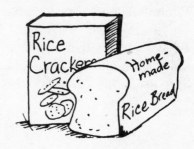

Beverages
(water—preferably
bottled,
filtered or distilled
Rose hips or peppermint
tea)

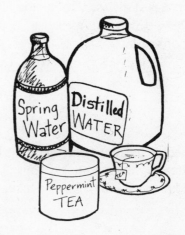

Miscellaneous
(fresh shelled unprocessed
nuts, seeds and oils—no
peanuts)

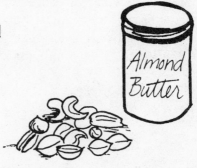

Vegetables:

White potatoes, Tomatoes, Sweet potatoes, Cabbage, Lettuce, Carrots, Squash, Asparagus, Cauliflower, Onions, Radishes, Beets, Celery, Green Peppers, Greens (beet, mustard, collards, kale, spinach, etc.), Cucumbers, Okra, Eggplant, Brussel Sprouts, Turnips, Avocado, Broccoli, Parsnips, Rutabaga.

Fruits:

Apples, Bananas, Grapes, Peaches, Pears, Kiwi, Pineapple, Prunes, Raisins, Cantaloupe, Watermelon, Strawberries, Figs, Dates, Cherries, Apricots, Coconut, Plums, Nectarines, Persimmons, Blackberries, Blueberries, Cranberries, Dewberries, Boysenberries, Raspberries, Loganberries.

Meats:

Beef, Chicken, Pork, Veal, Turkey, Lamb, Fish (trout, salmon, tuna sardines*, etc.), Clams, Lobster, Crab, Oysters, Shrimp, Squirrel, Rabbit, Quail, Duck, Goose, Game birds, Pheasant, Venison.

Bread:

Bake your own bread (since most commercial products contain wheat or rye). You can use oat or rice flours or tapioca, potato or arrowroot starch. Also get acquainted with non-grain alternatives such as amaranth, buckwheat and quinoa.

*Make sure the sardines are packed in sardine oil.

Beverages:

Bottled, distilled or filtered water (glass bottles only). (Fresh frozen orange juice is okay if orange juice isn't part of your regular diet.) Some herbed teas are okay if you aren't highly sensitive to yeasts and molds. I especially recommend rose hips or peppermint tea. (Plain Lipton's tea may be okay if it isn't part of your regular diet.)

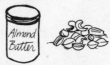

Miscellaneous:

Nuts . . . pistachios, English walnuts, black walnuts, hickory nuts, pecans, butternuts, almonds, Brazil nuts, chestnuts, hazel nuts, macadamias and pine nuts. (No peanuts.)

Honey and pure 100% maple syrup in moderation are okay— if you aren't yeast sensitive.

Safflower oil, sunflower oil, walnut oil, linseed oil, olive oil, canola oil.

Pure dairy butter (not margarine) may be okay. Most people with milk sensitivities are sensitive to milk proteins or intolerant to lactose. Such individuals may tolerate butter.

Foods You (or Your Child) Must Avoid

Milk, cheese, yogurt and other dairy products

Eggs or egg-containing foods

Foods containing wheat or rye

Foods containing corn

Foods containing sugar

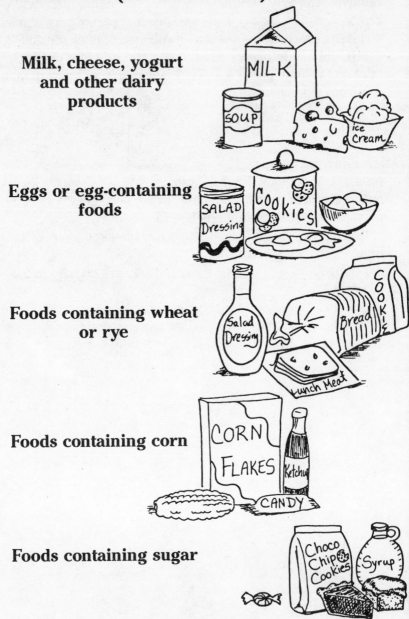

Chocolate and colas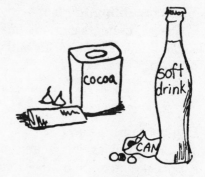

Yeast-containing foods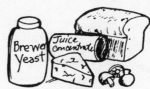

Coffee and alcohol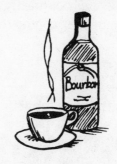

Soy, peanuts, beans and other legumes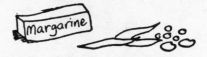

Coloring and additives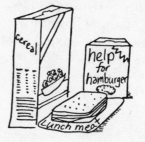

Milk-containing foods:

Cheese, butter, ice cream, margarines, breads, soups, cookies, candies, luncheon meats and other manufactured or processed foods.

Egg-containing foods:

Cakes, cookies, ice cream, pies, most pastas, salad dressings, pancake mixes and other manufactured or processed foods.

Wheat- and rye-containing foods:

Breads, cookies, crackers, most pastas, soups, cereals, candies, batters, luncheon meats, pancake mixes, salad dressings, gravies, and other commercially prepared foods.

Corn-containing foods:

Candies, breads, pastries, batters, cereals, ketchup, peanut butter, soft drinks, bacon and many other processed and refined products which contain corn oils, starches and sugars.

Sugar-containing foods:

Candies, soft drinks, cookies, ice cream, salad dressings, ketchup, and countless other packaged, processed and canned foods.

Chocolate- and Cola-containing foods:

Candies, snack foods, cereals, desserts, soft drinks.

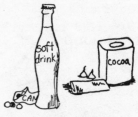

Yeast-containing foods

Brewers yeast, Bakers yeast, moldy cheeses, mushrooms, dried fruit, bottled and canned fruit juices and others. Raised breads and all fermented foods and beverages.

Coffee, tea & alcohol:

Coffee must be avoided. However, plain Lipton's tea, Rose hips, peppermint and other single ingredient herbed teas may be okay. Avoid all alcoholic beverages.

Legumes:

Green beans, lima beans, black-eyed peas, soy beans and other soy products, peanuts, tofu, carob and most gums. Many processed foods contain soy derivatives such as textured vegetable protein.

NOTE: To lessen your chances of making mistakes in planning, shopping and carrying out an elimination diet, avoid packaged and processed foods wherever possible. And when you use such foods, READ LABELS. Also try to avoid canned foods since many cans are lined with phenolic resins which cause symptoms in chemically sensitive individuals. Canned foods also contain yeast.

Foods You Can Eat For Breakfast

cantaloupe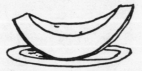

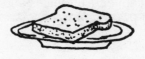 banana bread

fresh pineapple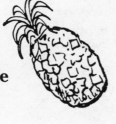

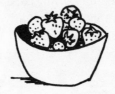 strawberries

rice cakes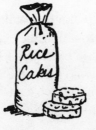

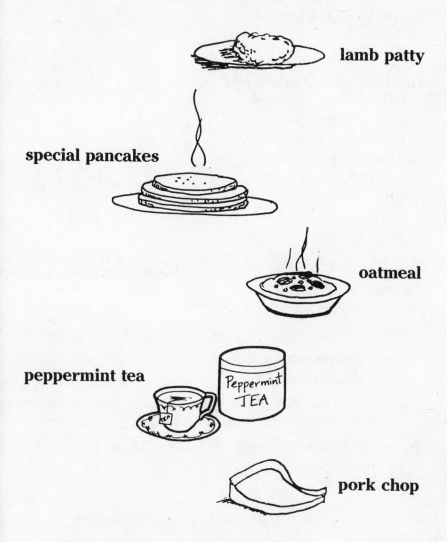

lamb patty

special pancakes

oatmeal

peppermint tea

pork chop

sliced potatoes

Breakfast Menus

Hot oatmeal (Quaker
   rolled oats), topped
   with chopped or
   shredded nuts.
   Moisten and sweeten
   with blended fruit
   (pineapple or
   banana).

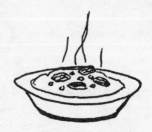

Banana.
*Buckwheat Banana
      Bread

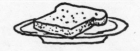

*Special pancakes made
   with buckwheat or
   amaranth

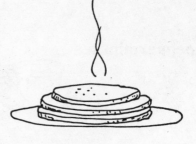

Fresh peaches (puréed)
   to top pancakes

Pecans

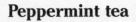

Peppermint tea

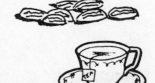

---

*See Recipes, pages 148–160.

Pork chops
Sweet potatoes, baked
Peaches, grapes,
   strawberries or other
   permitted fruit
Rice cakes or crackers

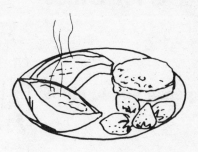

Fresh peaches or
   strawberries

*Fish (bake or poach in
   safflower oil, using
   oat or amaranth flour
   for batter). Sprinkle
   with almonds

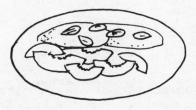

Sliced apples (or other
   fruit)

Ground beef (3 oz. or
   more)

Rice cakes

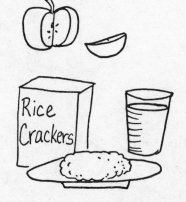

Ideas for Lunch

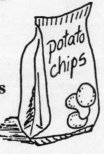

special potato chips

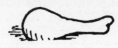
baked chicken

banana treat
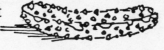

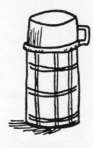
homemade chicken and rice soup

apple, pear
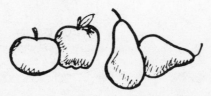

nuts (fresh shelled) (NO PEANUTS)

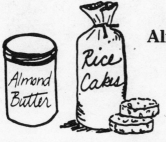 **Almond butter on rice crackers**

celery sticks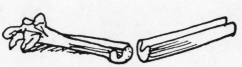

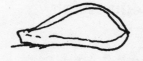 **pork chop**

grapes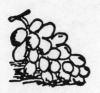

Lunch Menus

Hamburger patty, salt & pepper (no buns or "fixings")

Banana treat (banana, spread with almond butter, put halves together, and roll in ground almonds)

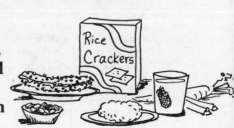

Carrot sticks

Rice crackers

Homemade chicken and rice soup*

Rice crackers

Grapes or other fresh fruit

Chicken leg baked (Use oat, amaranth or buckwheat flour for "breading".)

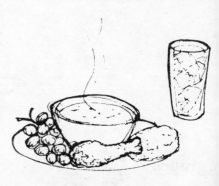

Peppermint tea

*See Recipes, pages 148–160.

Almond butter on rice
crackers

Celery sticks

Almonds

Apple (or other fresh
fruit)

Bottled water

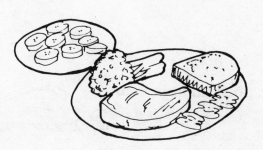

Pork chop

Steamed broccoli

Banana

English walnuts

Buckwheat bread

Tuna fish
(water-packed) on
rice crackers

Potato chips (made
with safflower or
cottonseed oil) which
contain no
additives

Plums or other fresh
fruit

Pecans

Rose hips tea

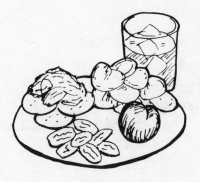

Suggestions for Supper

chicken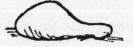

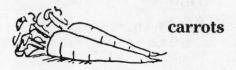 **carrots**

pork chop or lamb chop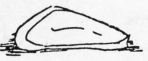

 **rice**

broccoli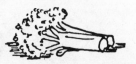

baked potato

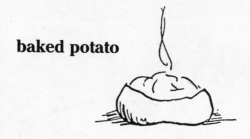

banana

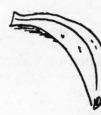

steak

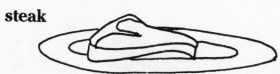

lettuce and tomatoes

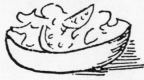

strawberries

Supper Menus

Lamb chop

Baked potato

Lettuce and tomato
   salad

Fresh pineapple

Rice crackers or cakes

Special boiled
   mayonnaise

Baked fish

Steamed kale

Sweet potato

Rice crackers

Cole slaw*

Dessert . . . mixed
   fruits covered with
   shredded coconut

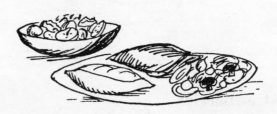

Oven-baked chicken*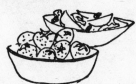
Baked sweet potato*
Carrots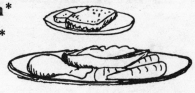
Mini rice cakes
Apple-nut salad on
    lettuce leaf
Strawberries

Broiled steak or baked
    red snapper
Baked potato
Broccoli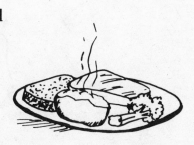
Buckwheat banana
    bread

Pork chop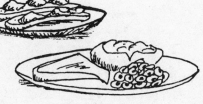
Baked potato
Brussel sprouts with
    lemon juice
Banana, almond butter
    salad*
Watermelon, cantaloupe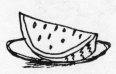
    (or other fruit)

Between Meal Snacks

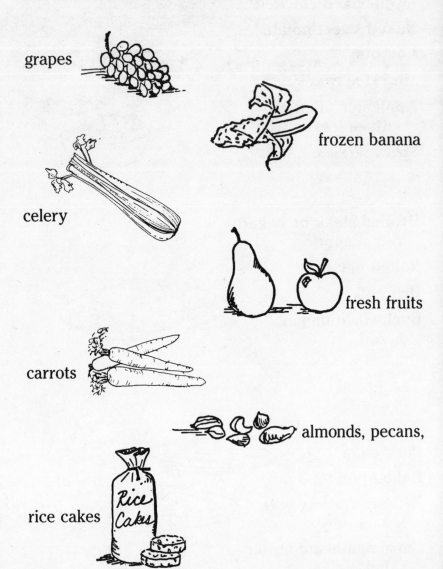

grapes

frozen banana

celery

fresh fruits

carrots

almonds, pecans,

rice cakes

SHOPPING TIPS FOR ELIMINATION DIET A

From Your Supermarket:

1. Stock up on all fresh fruits and vegetables (except corn, peas, beans and other legumes.)

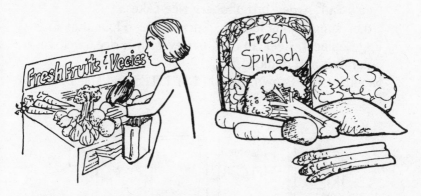

2. Buy chicken, beef, pork and fish including tuna canned in spring water and sardines packed in sardine oil. (Stay away from hot dogs, bacon, sausage, ham and luncheon meats since these products usually contain coloring and additives. Turkey and other poultry are sometimes injected with chemicals. Read labels.)
3. Other suggestions: Quaker rolled oats, Chico-San, Arden, Lundberg or other pure rice cakes, coconut in shell.

From Your Health Food Store:

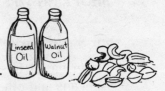

1. Unrefined sunflower, safflower, sesame, linseed or walnut oil.
2. Nuts in shell or additive-free nuts.

3. Chico-San, Arden or Lundberg rice cakes.
4. Other suggestions include: Ener-G Rice Flour and Ener-G Egg Replacer, steel cut oats, barley, brown rice, buckwheat, amaranth and quinoa.
5. Health Valley Brown Rice, FRUIT LITES and Oat Bran Hot Cereal.

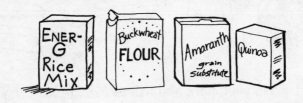

ELIMINATION DIET B
(Also known as the Rare Food or Cave Man Diet)

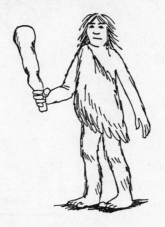

What is the "Cave Man Diet"? When and why should you try it? This term is used to attract your attention. It's also used to describe a *diet which avoids every food you eat more than once or twice a week.*

Here's why it may help you. Food sensitivities can be caused by any food, especially those you eat frequently. So, this diet gives you suggestions for eating nutritious and satisfying meals, consisting of foods you rarely eat. That's why I call it the Rare Food or Cave Man Diet.

In studying their patients with severe, long-standing health problems, some physicians use the Cave Man Diet initially. Others use it when their patients don't improve on Elimination Diet A.

Foods You (or Your Child) Can Eat

Meats*
(any but beef, chicken and pork)

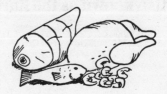

Grain Alternatives
(Amaranth, Buckwheat, Quinoa)

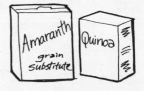

Fruits
(any but apples and citrus fruits)

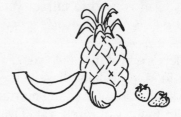

Nuts**
(filbert, Brazil nut, English walnut, almond, pecan)

 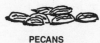

ALMONDS   PECANS

---

*Suggest wild game, duck or unusual fish or seafood.
**Also macadamia and pine nuts (pignolias).

Vegetables
(any but corn, white potato, tomato and legumes)

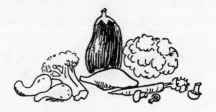

Safflower, Sunflower, Walnut, Olive or Canola oils

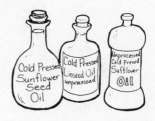

Beverages
(Mineral water, spring water)

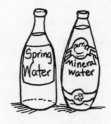

Vegetables:

Sweet Potatoes, Cabbage, Carrots, Squash (many varieties), Asparagus, Cauliflower, Celery, Garlic, Okra, Onions, Radishes, Greens (Beet, Mustard, Spinach, Collards, etc.), Cucumbers, Eggplant, Brussel sprouts, Kale, Avocado, Broccoli, Parsnips, Green peppers, Rutabaga, Jicama, Fennel, Leek, Turnips

Fruits:

Bananas*, Grapes*, Peaches, Pears, Pineapple, Kiwi, Papaya, Mangos, Melons (Watermelon, Cantaloupe, Honey Dew, Cranshaw), Cherries, Apricots, Coconut, Plums, Persimmons, Blackberries, Blueberries, Cranberries, Dewberries, Raspberries, Loganberries

Meats, Fish, Seafood, Poultry:

Turkey**, Fish***, Lamb, Shrimp, Deer, Rabbit, Duck, Goose, Oysters, Clams, Lobster, Crab, Squirrel, Pheasant, Frog legs, Quail, Scallops, Cornish hen

---

*The purpose of Diet B is to avoid any and every food you or your child eat more than once a week. Accordingly, if you love bananas, eliminate them. And if you snack regularly on grapes, eliminate them too. If you know of or detect sensitivity to any of the allowed foods eliminate those as well.

**Many commercial turkeys are basted with milk, corn or other additives and must be avoided on Elimination Diet B.

***Select unusual varieties of fish including grouper, orange roughy, or oreo dory.

Breads, Cakes, Crackers:

Because wheat, corn, rice, rye, oats, barley, millet and other grains are common causes of chronic allergy, and because all grains belong to the same "food family," *avoid all grains while on this diet.* (This means you must avoid the popular commercially available breads.) However, you can use the grain alternatives such as buckwheat*, amaranth and quinoa to make homemade flatbreads, pancakes and crackers. (See Recipes, pages 154–158.)

Beverages:

Bottled mineral water, distilled or spring water.

Miscellaneous:

Nuts (fresh shelled), untreated . . . pistachios, English walnuts, black walnuts, hickory nuts, pecans, butternuts, almonds, Brazil nuts, chestnuts, hazelnuts, pine nuts, macadamia nuts. (No peanuts.)

Safflower, walnut, olive, canola, sesame and sunflower oils.

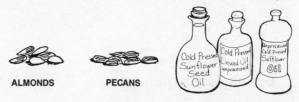

ALMONDS   PECANS

---

*Although buckwheat does not belong to the grain family, Elmer Cranton, M.D., Trout Dale, Virginia, recently commented, "Many grain sensitive people react to buckwheat." Thomas Stone, M.D. of Rolling Meadows, Illinois said, "People who are allergic to grains are nearly always sensitive to buckwheat—and to bananas too!" Based on these observations, amaranth and quinoa appear to be better choices for grain alternatives, especially during the first weeks of your Cave Man Diet.

Foods You (or Your Child) Must Avoid

milk, cheese, yogurt

egg

All grains
corn, wheat

citrus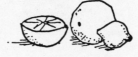

sugar

legumes
beans, peas, peanuts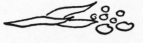

chocolate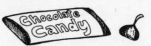

beef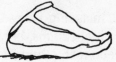

pork

apple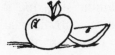

white potato

yeast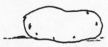

processed and packaged foods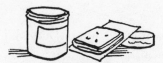

food coloring, additives, emulsifiers, preservatives

coffee, tea & alcohol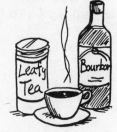

Milk-containing foods:

Milk and dairy products, including cheese, butter, ice cream, margarines, and yogurt, cream soups, breads, crackers, cookies, cakes, candies, luncheon meats, and other manufactured or processed foods.

Egg-containing foods:

Egg or any foods containing egg, including custards, cakes, cookies, ice cream, pies, macaroni, salad dressings, noodles, pancake mixes, and other manufactured or processed foods.

Grain-containing foods:

Wheat, corn, rye, barley, rice, and all other grains or foods containing grains. This includes all commercial breads, cookies, crackers, cereals, batters, luncheon meats, pancake mixes, candies and a wide variety of other packaged and processed foods.

Citrus:

Orange, grapefruit, lemon, and all foods containing citrus fruits or citric acid.

Sugar-containing foods:

Cane and beet sugars, including candies, cakes, sugar-coated cereals, ice cream, carbonated beverages, and a wide variety of processed and packaged foods which contain sugar. Sugar is hidden in dozens of other foods including catsup, pickles, relishes and salad dressings.

Legumes:

Peanuts, beans and peas of all kinds, including string beans, lima beans, soy beans, baked beans, green peas, field peas, black-eyed peas, carob and vegetable gums. Soy bean protein ("textured protein") is also hidden in a wide variety of manufactured foods.

Chocolate- & Cola-containing foods:

Avoid chocolate and cola drinks of all kinds; also all candies and other foods to which chocolate has been added.

Meats:

All forms of beef, pork and chicken, including luncheon meats, hot dogs, bacon, sausage and hamburger.

Fruits & Vegetables:

Baked potatoes, French fried potatoes, potato chips and any other food containing potato; tomato, corn, rice, orange, apple (including fresh, frozen or dried apples, apple juice or any foods containing apple flavoring) and any fruit or vegetable eaten more often than once a week.

Yeast-containing foods:

Breads, wine, vinegar, mushrooms, vitamins, condiments, dried fruits and many stored, frozen or canned foods including bottled or canned fruit juices.

Coffee, tea & alcohol:

All coffee and tea (including instant and caffeine free) products must be avoided. Also all alcoholic beverages.

Foods You Can Eat For Breakfast

lamb patty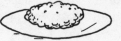

sweet potato slices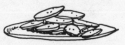

strawberries

 allowed nuts

pineapple chunks
sprinkled
with pecans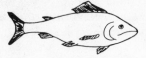

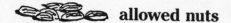 fresh fish

fresh melon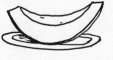

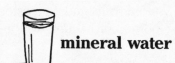 mineral water

sliced turkey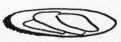

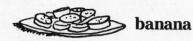 banana

Breakfast Menus

Lamb patty
Sliced bananas
Chopped pecans
Bottled mineral water

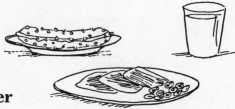

Fresh fish baked or
   broiled

Fresh pineapple

Shredded fresh coconut
   & chopped Brazil nuts
   (fresh shelled)

Bottled mineral water

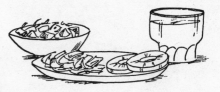

Turkey slices
Sweet potato slices
Fresh melon
Chopped nuts
Bottled mineral water

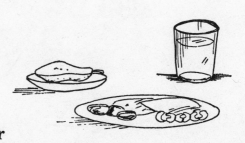

Ideas for Lunch

lamb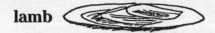

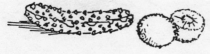 **banana treat or kiwi fruit**

pears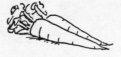

 almonds

carrots

shrimp and pineapple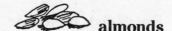

grapes

 shrimp salad

turkey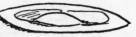

Lunch Menus

Slices of cold lamb
Sweet potato slices
Banana treat (split
  banana, spread with
  nut butter, put halves
  together, and roll in
  ground nuts)
Bottled mineral water

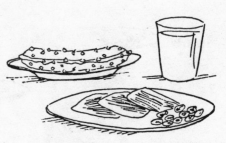

Broiled snapper
Wedge of cabbage, raw
  or steamed
Almonds
Pear

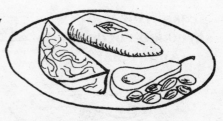

Shrimp salad made
  with chopped Brazil
  nuts, chopped celery
  and chopped raw
  carrots
Oil & lemon juice
  dressing
Almonds
Grapes

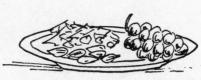

Suggestions for Supper

lamb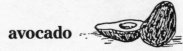

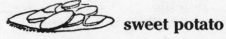 **sweet potato**

avocado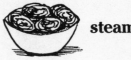

 steamed carrots

fresh fruit with shredded coconut (Ambrosia)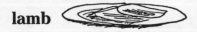

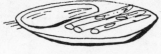 **asparagus and almonds**

baked fish

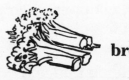 **broccoli**

banana

Supper Menus

Broiled shrimp on
  skewers with
  pineapple
Spinach
Baked squash
Fresh raspberries or
  other allowable fruit
  in season

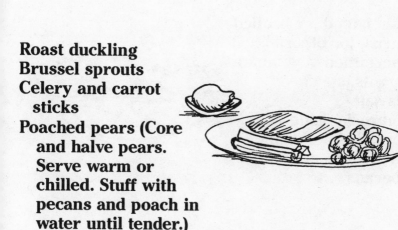

Roast duckling
Brussel sprouts
Celery and carrot
  sticks
Poached pears (Core
  and halve pears.
  Serve warm or
  chilled. Stuff with
  pecans and poach in
  water until tender.)

Pheasant
Baked potato
Vegetable medley
Fruit salad (bananas &
  grapes with shredded
  coconut on top)

Turkey
Baked sweet potato
Cauliflower, baked, or
  steamed
Sea salt
Sliced bananas, and
  chopped English
  walnuts

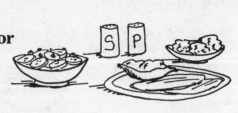

Fish, baked, or broiled
Squash (or other
  permitted vegetable)
Carrots, steamed
Sea salt
Ambrosia made with
  crushed pineapple,
  fresh coconut and
  pecans

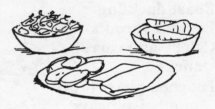

Lamb
Asparagus & almonds
Fruit & nut salad,
  containing pineapple,
  fresh strawberries (or
  sliced bananas),
  coconut and almonds.

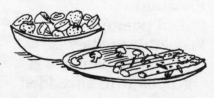

Snacks—At Work or After School

pineapple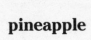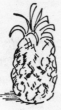

 mineral water

peaches

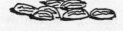 grapes

raw cauliflower, cucumbers or green peppers

 pecans

kiwi fruit

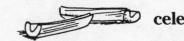 celery

allowed nuts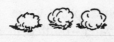

SHOPPING TIPS FOR ELIMINATION DIET B

From your supermarket:

1. Stock up on fresh fruits and vegetables *which you do not usually eat* such as asparagus, avocados, cherries, mangos, pears, pineapple, pomegranates, strawberries and sweet potatoes.

2. Buy lamb, fresh or fresh frozen turkey, fish, shrimp and other seafood.*
3. Other suggestions: Nuts in the shell 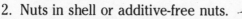 including almonds, brazil nuts, coconut and pecans. ALMONDS PECANS
4. Pure water (pure spring water, distilled water, mineral water—bottled in glass, or filtered water).**

From the health food store:

1. Sunflower, safflower, sesame, canola, linseed or walnut oils.
2. Nuts in shell or additive-free nuts.
3. Other suggestions: Bottled mineral water, almond nut butter.

Other rare and exotic foods can be ordered from a variety of sources some of which are listed on pages 92–95.

---

*Turkeys are often injected or treated with chemicals. Sulfites and other chemicals are sometimes added to retard spoilage right on the boat when caught.

**Most public waters are chemically contaminated. Filters can be purchased or obtained on lease. See the Yellow Pages of your phone book.

More Shopping Tips and Food Sources

More Shopping Tips*

1. Feature fresh foods or fresh frozen foods.
2. Avoid canned, packaged, processed or chemically-contaminated foods. (See pages 138–145.)

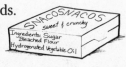

3. Avoid processed, smoked or cured meats, such as salami, wieners, bacon, sausage, hotdogs, etc., since they often contain milk, corn, sugar, food coloring and other additives.

4. If you must use a canned or packaged food, read the label carefully.

5. Avoid canned fruits packed in heavy or light syrup, since they contain cane or corn sugar. Instead, buy fruits packed in their own juices. Better still, use fresh fruits or fresh frozen fruits. (Check labels to make sure they do not contain sugar.)

6. Some fish are canned in vegetable oil. Since the oil may be of an unknown source, buy fresh fish or fish packed in water, or in its own oil.

---

*Some tips are appropriate for Diet A while others are useful for Diet B, and still others are helpful for both diets.

7. Most commercially available nuts are roasted in vegetable oil and contain additives. Accordingly, buy nuts in the shell, or shelled nuts which you know have not been dusted with a starch or otherwise treated (usually available from health food stores).

8. Most commercial frozen turkeys are injected with all kinds of things and are basted with milk or corn. You'll need to avoid them and buy turkey from other sources.

9. Use rice crackers for a bread substitute (read labels). Or bake your own bread using Ener-G rice flour*, or other special flour.

10. Use safflower, sunflower, sesame, olive, linseed or walnut oil in cooking or for salad dressings. (Combine with lemon juice.)

11. You can use 100% pure Carob powder as a substitute for chocolate. (Make sure it does not contain sugar or starch.)

12. Buy sea salt or canning salt, since some commercial salts contain corn starch. Don't get the kind that states that it "pours when it rains." This means chemicals have been added.

13. Buy grain alternatives, including amaranth, buckwheat and quinoa.

Food Sources

Cellu cereal-free baking powder; Cellu rice wafers, tapioca flour; Water packed fruits; Potato starch flour:
> *Chicago Dietetic Supply, Inc., LaGrange, IL 60525*

Caracoa carob powder:
> *El Molino Mills, P.O. Box 119, Pearl River, NY 10965*

*See Recipes, pages 148–160.

Rice cakes:
Arden Organic, 99 Pond Road, Asheville, NC 28806
Hain Pure Food Company, Inc., Los Angeles, CA 90061

Rice crackers (contain whole brown rice, sesame seeds & salt):
Chico San, Inc., 1144 West First Street, Chico, CA 95926

Potato chips (contain potato, safflower oil & salt, no additives):
Health Valley Natural Foods, Inc., 700 Union, Montebello, CA 90640

Sesame oil, safflower oil, sunflower oil:
Arrowhead Mills, Inc., Hereford, TX 79045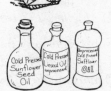

Nuts & Seeds:
Midwest Nut & Seed Company, Inc., 1332 W. Grand, Chicago, IL 60622

Ener-G rice mix; Ener-G egg replacer:
Ener-G Foods, Inc., P.O. Box 24723, Seattle, WA 98124

Unsweetened spreads (raspberry, strawberry & other fruits):
Westbrae Natural Foods, Berkeley, CA 94706

Rice Crunch Crackers, plain (Kitanihon Company):
Tree of Life, P.O. Box 1391, St. Augustine, FL 32084

Organic foods and exotic meats such as game & game birds of the U.S.A., and a few foreign animals:
Czimer Food, Inc., Rt. 1, Box 285, Lockport, IL 60441

Glass-canned natural Alaskan salmon with no seasonings or pre-servatives:
Briggs Way Company, Ugashik, AK 99683

Fresh fruits & vegetables:
Vita Green Farms, P.O. Box 878, 1525 W. Vista Way,
Vista, CA 92083

Persimmons, zapota, cherimoya, prickly pear, avocado & pomegranate:
> *Sam King, Alvarado Street, Fairmont, CA 94530*

Sweet potatoes:
Al Mueller, 233 Dade Avenue, Ferguson, MO 63135

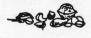

Nuts, especially pecans:
J. H. O'Neal, P.O. Box 565,
Donalsonville, GA 31745

Taro, mountain potato, yucca, boniata, apio root, ginger and fresh fish:
> *Del Farm Food Company, 4610 N. Clark Street, Chicago, IL 60600*

Bottled water, fruits and juices, vegetables, baked goods, dairy products, nuts, grains, flours, meats and seafoods:
> *Shiloh Farms, Sulphur Springs, AR 72768*

Cassave bread, *Malanga bread, *Lotus Bread, Amaranth bread, *Milo bread, White Sweet Potato Bread
  Ingredients: Flours above, distilled water, soda, calcium phosphate, salt—No oil*:
> *Special Foods, 9207 Shotgun Court (APD), Springfield, VA 22153, 703/644-0991, Mail order breads*

---

*Check with your local health food store. They may be able to supply some of the foods on this list. Also, see if you can obtain organically-grown foods—foods which are free of chemicals and insecticide spray (see also pages 137–146.)

Grains and grain products—Amaranth:
Walnut Acres, Inc., Penns Creek, PA 17682,
717/837-0601

Non-gluten amaranth seed and flour:
> *Post Rock Natural Grains, Route 1, Box 24 (APD),*
> *Luray, KS 67649, 913/648-2382*

Gelatin, agar:
> *Eden Foods, Inc., Clinton, MI 49236*

Quinoa flour and cereal:
> *Quinoa Corporation, P.O. Box 7114,*
> *Boulder, CO 80306, 800/237-2304*

Amaranth flour, puffed or whole seeds:
> *Nu-World Amaranth, Inc., P.O. Box 2202,*
> *Naperville, IL 60566, 312/369-6819*

QUESTIONS AND ANSWERS ABOUT ELIMINATION DIETS*

Q Headaches have bothered me for years. I'm also troubled by a year-round stuffy nose, recurrent belly aches and muscle aches. Tests and medicines of all kinds haven't really helped. I'm wondering if my symptoms are food related and I'd like to try an elimination diet. What foods should I eliminate?

A You'll need to eliminate your favorite foods. Here's why: The more of a food you eat, the greater are your chances of developing an allergy to the food. To make things easier for you I've prepared two diets. The first of these, Diet A (see pages 49–72), eliminates foods many people eat every day including:

milk and all dairy products; egg; wheat; corn, corn syrup and corn sweeteners; yeast; peas, beans, peanuts and other legumes; cane and beet sugar; orange and other citrus fruits; chocolate; food coloring and additives.

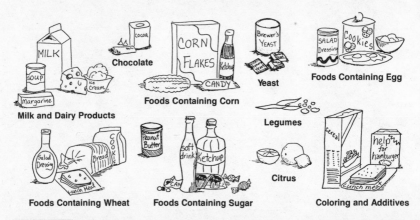

Milk and Dairy Products — **Chocolate** — **Foods Containing Corn** — **Yeast** — **Foods Containing Egg** — **Legumes** — **Foods Containing Wheat** — **Foods Containing Sugar** — **Citrus** — **Coloring and Additives**

---

*If you're sensitive to foods you're eating every day, chances are, you're also sensitive to tobacco, insecticides and other environmental chemicals. To gain maximum benefit from your diet detective work, do not smoke and avoid exposure to those who use tobacco. Also avoid perfumes, cosmetics, fumigants and other odorous chemicals (see also pages 138–145).

If your symptoms don't improve on Diet A, resume your usual diet for a few days, then try Diet B.

Q How do I get started on Diet A? What do I do first?
A Prepare menus and purchase foods you'll eat while on the diet. This requires careful planning.

Avoid commercially prepared or manufactured processed foods. Here's why: Such foods usually contain sugar, wheat, milk, corn, yeast, soy, food coloring and other ingredients which may be causing some of your symptoms.

Discuss the diet with your spouse and other family members. Study the list of permitted foods and feature those you and your family enjoy.

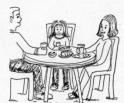

Q Tell me more about the diet.
A The diet is divided into two parts:

Part one: You eliminate a number of your usual foods to see if your symptoms improve or disappear.

Part two: You eat the foods again—one at a time—and note which foods cause your symptoms to return.

Q How will I know the diet is really making a difference?
A By keeping a record of your symptoms
   A. For three days (or more) before you begin your diet.
   B. While you're following the diet (5 to 7 days and sometimes longer).
   C. While you're eating the eliminated foods again—one at a time.

Q How will I feel on the diet?
A During the first two to four days on your diet, you're apt to feel irritable and hungry. And you won't feel satisfied even though you fill up on the permitted foods. You may feel restless and fidgety or tired and droopy.

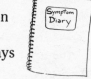

You may develop a headache or leg cramps. You may feel "mad at the world" because you aren't getting foods you crave—especially sweets. You may feel like a two pack a day smoker who has just given up the "weed." (People with hidden food allergies are usually addicted to the foods they're allergic to).*

Here's some good news. *If foods you've avoided are causing your symptoms, you'll usually feel better by the fourth, fifth or sixth day of your diet.* Almost always, you'll improve by the tenth day. Occasionally it will take two to three weeks before your symptoms go away.

Q If I improve on the diet, what do I do then? When and how do I return foods to my diet?

A *After you're certain that all or most of your symptoms are better and your improvement has lasted for at least 2 days, start eating the foods again—one food each day.* If you're allergic to a food you've eliminated, you should develop symptoms when you eat the food again.

Q What symptoms should I look for and how soon will I notice them?

A Usually, but not always, your main symptoms will reappear. In your case, you'd probably develop a headache or your nose would stuff up and you'd feel tired and depressed. However,

*Dr. Elmer Cranton comments: "If you substitute a non-allergic food of equal nutritional value for a frequently eaten food and feel cravings, you've confirmed the diagnosis of allergic addiction to that food. No matter how much you think you need the formerly eaten food, you will probably feel better, long term, without it!"

sometimes you'll notice other symptoms including some that haven't bothered you before including itching, coughing or urinary frequency.

Your symptoms will usually reappear within a few minutes to a few hours. However, some people may not notice a significant symptom until the next day. (Nearly always, if you avoid an allergy-causing food for a short period—five to twelve days—you'll develop symptoms promptly when you eat the food again. By contrast, if you avoid a food for three or more weeks, your sensitivity will usually lessen and your symptoms won't appear until you eat the food two or three days in a row.)

Q When I eat a food again, does it make any difference what form the food is in?

A Yes! Yes! Yes! Add the food in pure form. For example, when you eat wheat, use pure whole wheat (obtainable from a health food store) rather than bread, since bread contains milk and other ingredients. If you're adding milk, use whole milk rather than ice cream since ice cream contains sugar, corn syrup and other ingredients.

Here are suggestions for returning foods to your diet:

Egg: Eat a soft or hard boiled egg or eggs scrambled or fried in pure safflower or sunflower oil.

Citrus: Peel an orange and eat it or drink fresh squeezed orange juice.

Yeast: Use Brewer's yeast tablets, Baker's yeast and mushrooms. If you pass the milk challenge, eat some moldy cheese.

Wheat: Get 100% pure whole wheat from your health food store. Add water and cook for 20 to 25 minutes. Add sea salt if you wish. Eat it straight or add sliced bananas or strawberries. (If you want to "wet" the cereal, you can put the fruit in a blender with a little water and pour it on the cereal like milk or cream.)

If you don't like hot cereals, you can use shredded wheat. However, shredded wheat contains the additive BHT which may cause symptoms. So a pure wheat product without additives is better.

Food coloring: Buy a set of McCormicks or French's dyes and colors. Put a half teaspoon of several colors in a glass. Add a teaspoon of the mixture to a glass of water and sip on it. If you show a reaction, you'll later need to test the various food dyes separately. Red seems to be the most common offender.

Legumes: Eat some peanuts, peas, string beans, lima beans, soy beans, black-eyed peas or other legumes. Get peanuts in shell or soy from a health food store. Some people who are allergic to peanuts or soy will be sensitive to all legumes while others may tolerate some legumes and may not tolerate others.

Chocolate: Use Baker's cooking chocolate or Hershey's cocoa powder. You can sweeten it with a little liquid saccharin. (Sweeta or Fasweet) Eat the powder with a spoon or add it to water and make a chocolate flavored drink.

Corn: Use fresh corn on the cob, pure corn syrup, grits or hominy. Eat plain popcorn. Don't use microwave popcorn because it contains other ingredients.

Sugar: Get plain cane sugar. Perhaps the easiest way to do this is to eat some sugar lumps or add the sugar to a glass of water. Do the same with beet sugar.

Milk: Use whole milk.

Q I think I understand what you want me to do. However, a few points aren't clear. Please go over them again.

A Okay, here they are:

1. Carefully review all your instructions. Plan ahead. Don't start your diet the week before Christmas, Thanksgiving or some other holiday—and don't start it when you're travel-

ing or visiting friends or relatives. Ask—even beg—other family members to help you and to cooperate. Study your instructions and purchase the foods you'll need. Keep a diary of your symptoms for at least three days before you begin your diet.

Remain on the diet until you're absolutely certain your symptoms have improved. Remember that your symptoms are apt to worsen the first 48 to 72 hours on the diet.

Usually, you'll feel better by the fourth or fifth day although some people won't notice a significant change until they've followed the diet for seven to ten days—occasionally longer. Still other individuals with a hidden food allergy won't show a lot of improvement until they've avoided an offending food for two or three weeks. However, such people are the exception.

2. If you don't feel significantly better in ten to fourteen days*, start eating your usual foods—even pig out. If your symptoms worsen (including your headache, fatigue, irritability or stuffiness), chances are they're food related and you'll have to do further detective work to identify the troublemakers.

3. If you improve on the diet, return the eliminated foods one at a time and see if you develop symptoms. Here's how you go about it.
   A. Add the foods you least suspect first. Save the foods you think are causing your problems until last. Remember, you're apt to be allergic to your favorite foods.
   B. If you have no idea what foods are causing your symptoms, here's a suggested order for returning foods to your diet.

---

*Your failure to improve substantially on an elimination diet may be related to other offending substances in your living and work environment (exhaust fumes, paint fumes, insecticide sprays, carpet odors, etc.). Accordingly, before beginning your diet, clean up your environment (see pages 138–145).

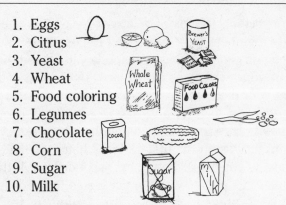

1. Eggs
2. Citrus
3. Yeast
4. Wheat
5. Food coloring
6. Legumes
7. Chocolate
8. Corn
9. Sugar
10. Milk

4. Eat a small portion of the eliminated foods for breakfast. If you show no reaction, eat more of the food for lunch and for supper and between meals too.*

5. *Keep the rest of your diet the same while you're carrying out the challenges.* Here's an example: Suppose you eat wheat on the first day of your diet and show no reaction. Does this mean you can continue to eat wheat? No. Eat wheat only on the day of the challenge and don't eat it again until you've tested all the foods and the diet has been completed.

6. If you show no symptoms after adding a food the first day, add another food the second day, eating all you want— *unless you show a reaction.*

7. If you think you develop symptoms when you add a food but aren't certain, eat more of the food until your symptoms are obvious. But don't make yourself sick.

    If you show an obvious reaction after eating a food such as stuffiness, cough, irritability, nervousness, drowsiness, headache, stomach ache, flushing or wheezing, don't eat more of that food. Wait until the reaction subsides (usually 24 to 48 hours) before you add another food.

---

*If a person suffers from severe asthma, hives or swelling, the food challenges should be supervised by a physician and carried out in his office or clinic.

If a food really bothers you, shorten the reaction by taking a teaspoonful of "soda mixture" (2 parts baking soda and 1 part potassium bicarbonate—your pharmacist can fix up this mixture for you). Or dissolve two tablets of Alka Seltzer Gold* in a glass of water and drink it. A saline cathartic such as Epsom salts will also shorten your reaction by eliminating the offending foods from your digestive tract rapidly.

Q Thank you for those explanations. They make sense. But while we're discussing diets, lets go ahead and talk about Diet B.

A I call Diet B the "Rare Food" or "Cave Man" Diet. On this diet you'll eliminate all the foods listed on Diet A. In addition, you must avoid beef, chicken, pork, white potato, tomato, rice, oats, coffee, tea and any food or beverage you consume more than once a week.

For example, if you eat bananas and apples daily or several times a week, add them to the list of the foods you eliminate. If you snack on pecans, avoid them. But if you rarely eat a food, you need not leave it out of your diet.

Q I can see that this diet is a truly comprehensive one. Would I be able to get enough to eat?

A Yes. Although early on you'd probably suffer food cravings which we've already discussed. But you can eat as much as you want of the allowed foods. So you get plenty of nutrition. My purpose in prescribing the Cave Man Diet is to avoid foods you usually eat. But to repeat—as difficult as this diet seems to be, it provides you with a variety of wholesome foods (see list on pages 73–77). Do you think you'll be able to carry out this Diet B?

---

*Alka Seltzer Gold contains no aspirin.

Q Yes—I can do anything I have to do. But let me repeat your instructions so I can be certain I understand them.

If I feel Diet A hasn't given me the answers I'm looking for, you're suggesting I try Diet B.* On this diet, I eliminate all the foods on Diet A plus pork, beef, chicken, potato, rice, oats and any food I eat more than once a week. So I'll have to eliminate twenty or more foods?

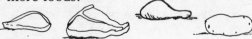

A That's right.

Q How about returning these foods to my diet? Do I add one food a day?

A That's one way to do it. However, it would take you three or four weeks to complete the diet.

Q That's a long time. And it would be hard for me to hold the line and keep from cheating. Is there another way to do Diet B in less time?

A Yes. Carry out the elimination phase of the diet until your symptoms improve, just as we've already discussed. However, if you improve promptly (as, for example, in 4 or 5 days), you can begin returning the foods to your diet sooner. You can also shorten the period you'll have to stay on the diet by adding the foods you've eliminated four times a day.

Q How would I do this? Please explain.

A After your improvement is convincing and you've continued to feel better for at least 48 hours, add a single food—such as orange—for breakfast. But before you add the food, take a few

---

*Some physicians advise their patients to begin their diet detective work with Diet B. Still other physicians begin with a four- or five-day fast.

For individuals with severe and incapacitating allergies, some physicians use an even more comprehensive elimination diet program. Rather than giving a person regular foods, they give them a special non-allergic protein mixture called Vivonex for five to seven days until their symptoms subside and then they return the eliminated foods to their diet.

minutes to make an inventory of your symptoms.* Think about how you feel. Does your head hurt? Are you tired? Is your nose stopped up? Do you have a burning in your stomach or aching in your legs? *It's important for you to "tune in" on symptoms that are present before eating the food.* If you fail to do this, you're apt to blame symptoms that are already present on the food you're testing.

After you've finished your symptom inventory, eat the orange. If no new symptoms develop, wait fifteen minutes and eat another orange, and then a third. If no symptoms develop, oranges aren't causing your problems.

Wait four hours, then introduce a second food (such as rice). Follow the same procedure that you followed in testing the orange. If this food causes no reaction, in another four hours, try a third food (such as baked chicken). Then eat a fourth food an hour before bedtime.

So each day you'll be eating four foods. By doing this you'll reduce the "adding back" phase of your diet from three weeks to seven to ten days.

Q Would that work as well?

A Perhaps. Such a rapid addition of foods would have several advantages. One of these would be completing Diet B in less time—two weeks rather than three more weeks. Another advantage relates to the peculiarities of a "hidden" food allergy.

Q Could you explain?

A I'll try. If you avoid a food you're allergic to for a week and then eat it again, it'll nearly always cause a reaction. But if you avoid it for two, three or more weeks, the level of your allergy may "die down" (see page 120) so that you may

---

*Counting your pulse before and after you eat a food may also help you determine a food reaction. A pulse acceleration of six to eight beats following a food challenge is usually significant.

show little reaction when you eat it again, especially if you consume only a small amount.

Q From what you've told me, I believe it'll be best for me to add one food four times a day. Will that be okay?

A Yes. I feel that's the best way.

Q Okay, now that's settled, I'd like your suggestions for getting my family to cooperate.

A Plan the diet carefully. Discuss it with other family members ahead of time. Where possible, feature foods all family members will eat (although they may want other foods to keep them satisfied and happy). Don't worry if your diet is limited. Even if you lose several pounds it won't hurt you and you'll soon regain them.

Q Can I follow the diet at work?

A Yes, if you "brown bag" it. If you're invited out to dinner, tell your host or hostess what you're doing and eat before you go or decline the invitation and ask for a raincheck.

Q Is it best to start with Diet A? Or would you recommend Diet B first? Doing Diet B might save me time and trouble.

A Sometimes I recommend Diet A for my patients and sometimes I recommend Diet B. *It depends on how the patient feels about it and how severe and long lasting his symptoms are.* However, in most patients I recommend Diet A.

Here's why: Most food sensitive people improve on Diet A and Diet A is easier to follow than Diet B. It eliminates many of the major food troublemakers. Yet, it allows a person to eat pork, chicken, potatoes, apples and other foods which he likes but which he doesn't eat every day. And the rest of your family can eat the same diet. This makes things easier.

Q When, why and under what circumstances should I try Diet B?

A As I've already indicated, it depends on many different things.

For example, although I've found that milk, wheat, corn, yeast, sugar, egg, chocolate, legumes and food additives are the most common troublemakers, *any food can cause a reaction.*

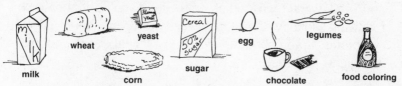

milk   wheat   yeast   corn   sugar   egg   legumes   chocolate   food coloring

So even if you improve when you remove these foods from your diet, you may continue to show symptoms because beef, pork, chicken, apple, potato, tomato, banana, oats or other foods may be causing some of your symptoms. *The only way you can tell if these foods bother you is to eliminate them from your diet and see if your symptoms improve.* Then you can eat the foods again and see if your symptoms return.

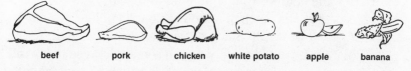

beef   pork   chicken   white potato   apple   banana

Q I think I understand. But to make sure, let me repeat your instructions. You want me to do Elimination Diet A for seven to ten days keeping a record of my symptoms for three days *before* I start the diet. I continue to record my symptoms for the seven to ten day elimination phase of the diet. Then after I'm sure my symptoms have improved, I eat the foods again, one at a time, to see which foods bother me and which foods do not. I continue my records.

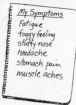

My Symptoms
Fatigue
foggy feeling
stuffy nose
headache
stomach pain
muscle aches

A That's right.

Q Suppose I complete the diet and note obvious reactions to a couple of foods, yet, there are other foods I'm not sure about—what do I do then?

A Keep the foods which cause reactions out of your diet indefinitely. Retest the foods you're uncertain about. Here's one way you can do this. Eat the suspected food several days in a row, as for example, Friday, Saturday, Sunday, Monday and Tuesday. Eliminate the food on Wednesday, Thursday, Friday, Saturday and Sunday and then load up on the food you've eliminated the following Monday. If you're allergic to it you should develop symptoms. If you show no symptoms, chances are you aren't allergic to that food.

Mon. Tue. Wed. Thu. Fri.

| 1 | 2 | 3 | 4 | 5 |

Q I think I understand but suppose I show a reaction when I eat wheat, egg or when I drink milk. Does this mean I'll always be allergic to these foods?

A Yes, to some degree. Your symptoms will nearly always return if you consume as much of a food as you did before you began your diet. However, if you avoid a food you're allergic to for several months, you'll usually regain some tolerance to it. And you may not develop symptoms unless you eat it several days in a row.

Q How do I find out?
A By trial and error.

Q I'm not sure I understand—please explain.
A I'll do my best. When you avoid a food you're allergic to for several months, you'll generally lose some of your allergy to the food (like a fire that dies down).

For example, if you're bothered by a stuffed up nose, headache and fatigue while drinking a quart of milk a day, you may

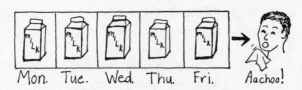

Mon. Tue. Wed. Thu. Fri. Aachoo!

be able to eat yogurt or cheese occasionally after you've eliminated milk from your diet for several months. However, suppose you eat milk-containing foods after you've avoided them for several months and show no reaction. In such a situation you may say to yourself, "The yogurt and cheese didn't bother me so maybe milk allergy isn't one of my problems. But if you start drinking milk or eating dairy products every day, within a few days or weeks some of your symptoms will return. Before you know it, you'll develop the same health problems you had before you eliminated the milk.

Sometimes, though, it takes even longer for your symptoms to recur and you may not connect them to the food.

Q I think this point is clear but why does a food bother me on some occasions and not on others. For example, I've heard of people who became congested when they drank milk in the winter but who could drink it in the summer without showing any symptoms.

A It has to do with the *"allergic load"* or *concomitant allergies*. Along with other physicians interested in food allergy, I have found that allergic individuals may tolerate foods in the summer which they can't eat in the winter.

Part of the problem relates to chilling. Also, winter time furnaces which stir up dust and dry out the respiratory membranes may lessen a person's resistance and make him more susceptible to winter time infections and allergies.

In addition, during the winter time, you spend more time indoors. Windows and doors are usually closed so there is less ventilation. Accordingly, disease-producing germs are more prevalent. Other factors include the household and office indoor air pollutants (tobacco smoke, perfumes, janitorial sup-

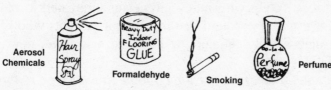

Aerosol Chemicals   Formaldehyde   Smoking   Perfumes

plies and other odorous chemicals). Cold weather, dust, cold germs and chemicals plus food allergies, cause many winter time health problems.

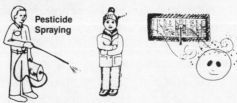

Pesticide Spraying

Q Do other allergies such as hayfever due to grass or bronchitis due to house dust mites or cat dander have anything to do with the amount of an allergy-causing food I can eat?

A Yes. The more allergy troublemakers you're exposed to, the greater are your chances of developing an allergic illness. For example, let's suppose you're allergic to milk, corn, chocolate, spring grass and house dust mites. Yet, you aren't severely allergic to any one of these substances.

Accordingly, you may play golf in the spring without being bothered by hay fever and you may be able to eat an occasional piece of cornbread or chocolate without symptoms. But if you eat a sack of popcorn, a candy bar and drink a chocolate milk shake on the same day (after cutting the grass), you may become irritable and nervous and develop nasal congestion or bronchitis.

Q I'm beginning to understand more about hidden food allergies. But suppose I'm allergic to egg and I avoid egg for three months. Then I eat an egg for breakfast and it doesn't bother me. How will I know how much and how often I can eat egg in the future?

A I'm glad you asked. It'll give me a chance to talk about a rotated diet. Along with many physicians interested in hidden food allergies, I've found that my allergic patients who rotate their diets usually get along well and develop fewer new food allergies.

Rotating a diet means eating a food only once every four to seven days. For example, if you're allergic to egg and after avoiding it for several months you eat an egg and it doesn't bother you, you can try eating an egg once a week and see if you tolerate it. You can do the same with other foods. (See also pages 134–135.)

S	M	T	W	T	F	S
1	2	3	4	5	6	7
8	9	10	11	12	13	14
15	16	17	18	19	20	21
22	23	24	25	26	27	28
29	30	31				

EGG DAY

Q Aren't some foods "kin" to each other—like chicken and egg, wheat and corn or milk and beef? Is a person who is allergic to one food more apt to become sensitive to foods in the same "family?"

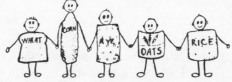

A The answer to both of your questions is "yes." Foods are "kin" to each other. Familiar food families include the grain family, citrus family and the legume family (peas, peanuts, beans and soybeans). While there are many exceptions, people who are sensitive to one food in a family are more apt to be sensitive— or become sensitive—to another food in the family, especially if they eat a lot of it.

I've found that wheat sensitive patients are apt to become sensitive to all other grains—especially if they eat them repeatedly or in quantity. Although I permit rice and oats on Diet A, if you find you're allergic to wheat or corn, experiment further with your diet to see if other grains cause reactions.

If you're allergic to grains, here's another suggestion: Go to your health food store and get some quinoa, amaranth and buckwheat. You can make bread and other grain-like products from these grain alternatives. Yet, they aren't "kin" to the grains.*

Now for a word on milk and beef. Most milk sensitive individuals seem to be able to eat steak and hamburger without a reaction. However, because cow's milk and beef come from the same animal, if you're allergic to milk, avoid beef for a week, then add it back and see what happens. If you're allergic to egg, limit your intake of chicken to a serving every four to seven days.

Is there anything else you'd like to know—anything at all?

Q Nothing I can think of at the moment—my head is spinning. Do you have further suggestions?

A Read, review and study all the instructions I've given you. When you've finished, you'll find that detecting your hidden food allergies won't be as hard as you thought it would be.

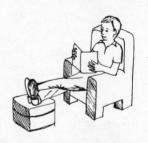

---

*See Recipes, pages 148–160. For more information on amaranth and quinoa, get a copy of Marge Jones' books, THE ALLERGY SELF-HELP COOKBOOK (Rodale Press) and AMARANTH & QUINOA . . . SUPER-FOODS OF THE AZTEC & INCA INDIAN. Marge also publishes a newsletter, MASTERING FOOD ALLERGIES. For more information, write to MAST Enterprises, Inc., 2615 North 4th St., Suite 677, Couer d'Alene, Idaho 83814.

Parables About Allergy

Introduction

Confucius say, "A journey of a thousand miles starts with one step." And overcoming your allergies, like the journey Confucius was talking about, requires many steps. Maybe not a thousand, but many.

And Dr. Susan Dees of Duke University, in talking about allergies some years ago, said in effect, "The more the allergic person knows about himself and the things he's sensitive to, and the more he knows about allergies and how they affect him, the better are his chances of overcoming them."

To help you understand more about allergies, especially food allergies, study the parables in the next few pages. Each one illustrates one or more important principles about allergy.

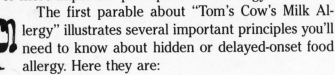 The first parable about "Tom's Cow's Milk Allergy" illustrates several important principles you'll need to know about hidden or delayed-onset food allergy. Here they are:

(a) Hidden food allergies are caused by foods you eat every day. When you eliminate them, your symptoms will usually clear up within a week.

(b) Then if you eat the foods again, following this short period of elimination, your symptoms will return.

(c) However, if you eliminate a food troublemaker for several months, you'll usually regain some tolerance to the food.

(d) After regaining tolerance, you can eat the food occasionally (such as every 4 to 7 days) without causing symptoms.

(e) Yet, if you eat a lot of the food every day, your tolerance will break down and your symptoms will return.

The second parable about Maria helps you to understand the concept of "allergy load." Your allergy symptoms may be caused by many different substances (including foods, pollens, house dust, molds, animal danders and emotional stress).

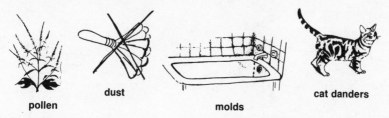

pollen   dust   molds   cat danders

In addition, you may be sensitive to tobacco smoke and chemical fumes which increase your allergic load. Finally, chilling and infection may also increase your chances of developing allergic symptoms.

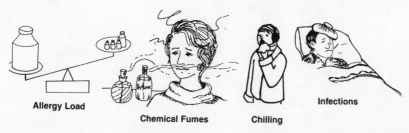

Allergy Load   Chemical Fumes   Chilling   Infections

If you understand Maria's story and identify your allergy troublemakers and keep them under control, you'll have a better chance of staying well.

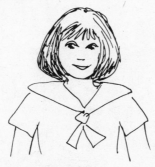

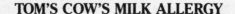

TOM'S COW'S MILK ALLERGY

When Tom was three months old he developed a scaly rash on his cheek.

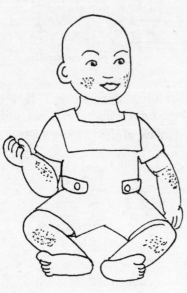

By the age of five months, the rash spread to other parts of his body. Ointments and creams didn't help.

When Tom was six months old, his mother took him off his cow's milk formula. His rash went away.

Two weeks later, Tom drank a few ounces of milk and the rash returned—worse than ever.

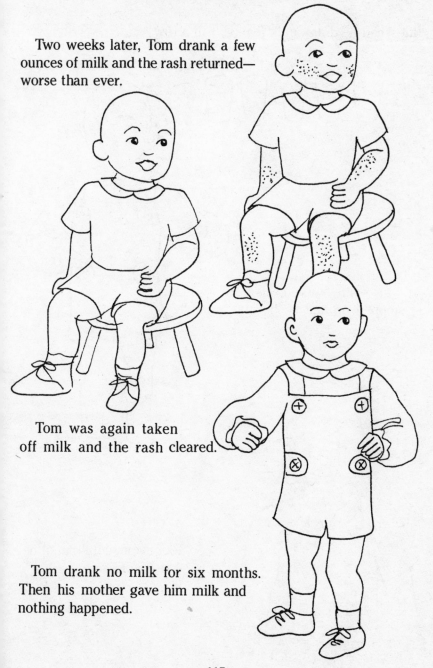

Tom was again taken off milk and the rash cleared.

Tom drank no milk for six months. Then his mother gave him milk and nothing happened.

But when he drank milk five days in a row

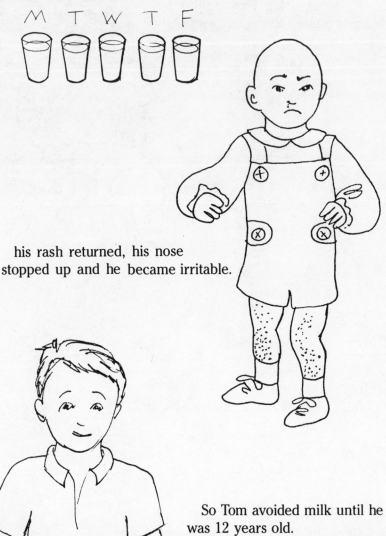

his rash returned, his nose
stopped up and he became irritable.

So Tom avoided milk until he
was 12 years old.

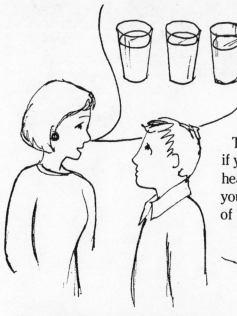

Then his teacher said, "Tom if you want to make an A in health on your report card, you must drink three glasses of milk each day."

Tom liked the milk and he felt fine, but after a month he began to complain of fatigue, headache, belly aches and muscle aches.

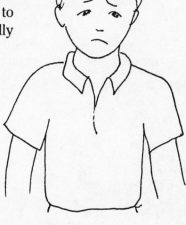

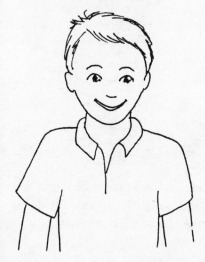

When Tom stopped drinking milk, his symptoms went away.

Now at the age of 35 Tom can drink milk or eat cheese or ice cream once a week and it doesn't bother him.

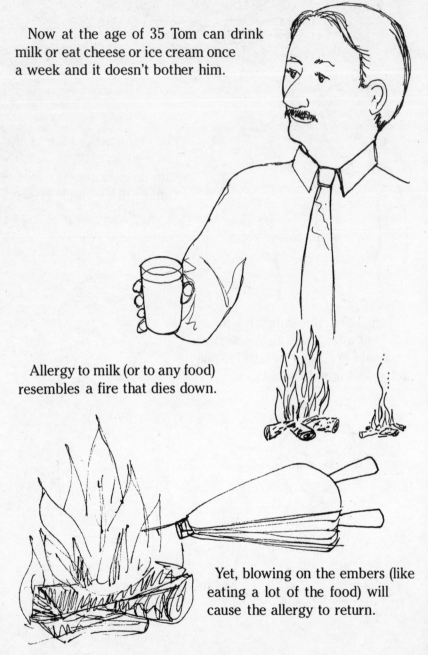

Allergy to milk (or to any food) resembles a fire that dies down.

Yet, blowing on the embers (like eating a lot of the food) will cause the allergy to return.

THE STORY OF MARIA

Maria is an allergic person and like most people with allergies, she's sensitive to many things that she eats, breathes or touches.

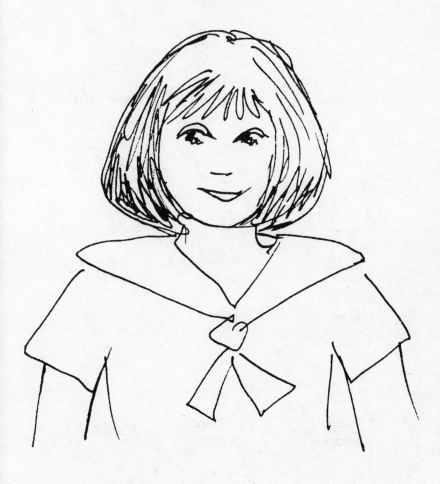

In addition, things other than allergens contribute to her symptoms.

The different troublemakers resemble weights.

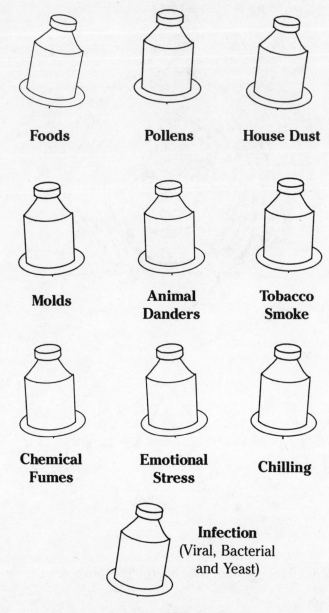

Foods   **Pollens**   **House Dust**

Molds   **Animal Danders**   **Tobacco Smoke**

Chemical Fumes   **Emotional Stress**   **Chilling**

Infection
(Viral, Bacterial and Yeast)

Yet, in spite of her allergies, Maria enjoys excellent health and feels good most of the time.

Here's why: She avoids the things that bother her so that her resistance is usually greater than her load of troublemakers. Here are examples:

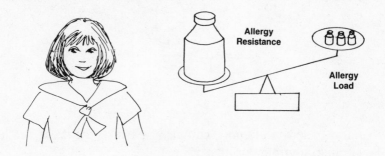

Although Maria was allergic to milk during infancy and childhood, she can eat yogurt or cheese once or twice a week without developing symptoms.

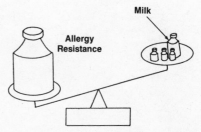

And she develops few symptoms in the spring if she avoids milk products and doesn't play golf when the pollen count is high.

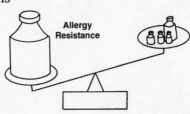

But if Maria consumes more dairy products when the trees are budding, her allergy load outweighs her resistance and she experiences more symptoms.

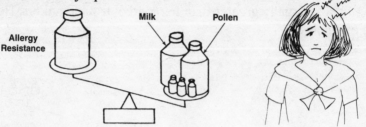

Maria's allergy tolerance can also be overcome if she drinks a lot of milk anytime during a year.

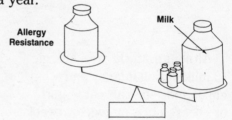

Or dust collects in her room, her cat sleeps on the foot of the bed, she's drinking milk and is exposed to tobacco smoke.

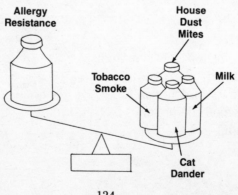

It can also be overcome in other ways.

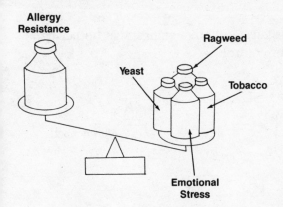

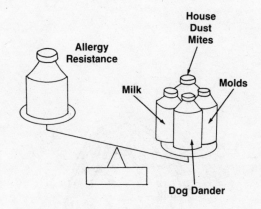

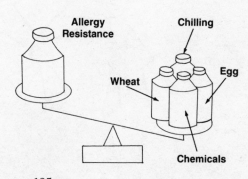

The best way for Maria (or any allergic person) to remain well is to—

1. Identify the allergens (and other things) that bother her.
2. Keep them under control.

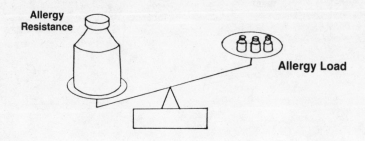

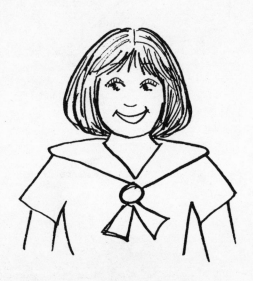

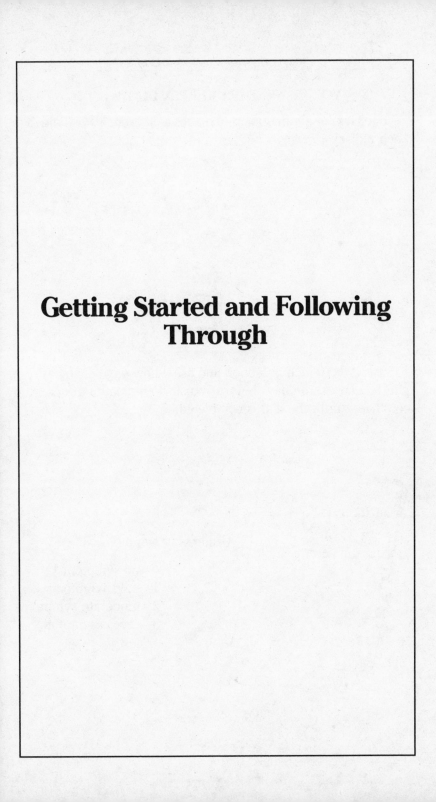

Getting Started and Following Through

YOU'LL NEED TO KEEP A DIARY . . . .

To tell if your elimination diet makes a difference, you'll need to keep a diary.

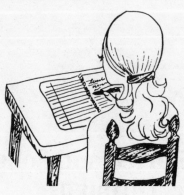

Buy an 8x10 inch notebook and use a new page each day. Begin the diary three days before you start eliminating foods. And continue it until the diet is completed.

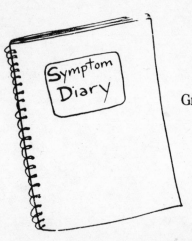

Grade your symptoms:

        0—no symptoms
        1—mild symptoms
        2—moderate symptoms
        3—severe symptoms

Here are examples: If you sniff or your nose runs all the time, put "2" in the respiratory column for each period during the 24-hours.

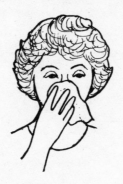

If you complain of a bad headache on arising each day, which gradually disappears by lunch time, put a "3" in the headache column "before breakfast," a "2" in the morning column, and put a "0" in the headache column for the rest of the day.

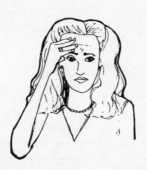

At the bottom of the page, list the foods you eat each day.
By keeping this diary, you can usually tell which foods . . . if any . . . are causing your complaints.

SYMPTOM AND DIET DIARY

SYMPTOMS	TIME OF DAY				
	Before Breakfast	After Breakfast	After Lunch	After Supper	During Night
Tired or Drowsy					
Irritable or Overactive					
Headache					
Respiratory (stuffy nose, cough, etc.)					
Digestive (belly ache, nausea, etc.)					
Muscle and joint symptoms					
Other					

	Breakfast	Morning	Lunch	Afternoon	Supper	Evening
WHAT YOU ATE TODAY						

STICKING TO YOUR DIET

An elimination diet could change your life. Approach it positively. Plan the diet carefully and execute it precisely (remember, it's a scientific study). Here are suggestions that will increase your chances of succeeding.

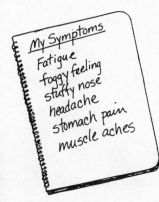

On the first page, write down a list of the symptoms that bother you.

Then stop a minute and think about really feeling good.

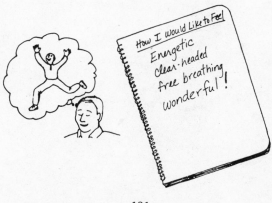

Enter the date you'll begin keeping your diary (while you're still eating your usual food).

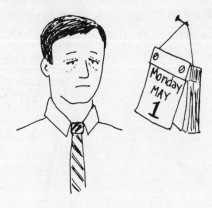

Write down the date you'll begin your diet (at least three days after you start keeping your diary).

Enter a date seventeen days after you begin your diet. (It usually takes seventeen days to eliminate the foods, feel better and add them back.)

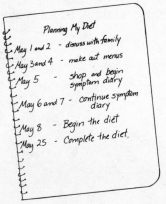

Planning My Diet

May 1 and 2 - discuss with family

May 3 and 4 - make out menus

May 5 - shop and begin symptom diary

May 6 and 7 - continue symptom diary

May 8 - Begin the diet

May 25 - Complete the diet

Discuss the diet with your spouse (or a friend or a business associate). Tell him/her of your determination. Make a public commitment.

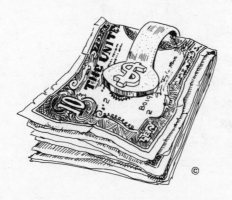

If your friend says, "I don't believe you'll stick to that diet," ask her to make a bet with you. (It needn't be a lot of money.)

Or you could say, "If I cheat on my diet, I'll give you a dollar. If I cheat more than once, I'll give you five dollars. If I don't complete the diet, I'll give you ten dollars."

You can work out a different agreement with your spouse and you might say, "Will you give me a dollar (or five dollars) each day I stick to my diet? If I complete it without cheating, I'll deserve a bigger reward. What will you offer?"

There are many different ways you can set up a behavior modification plan. Such a plan should enable you—

1. To have a positive mental image of what you're going to do.
2. To receive a reward for carrying out the diet successfully.

A Rotated Diet Helps

Variety is the spice of life . . . and a rotated diet will help you prevent and treat your hidden food allergies . . . and enjoy good health.

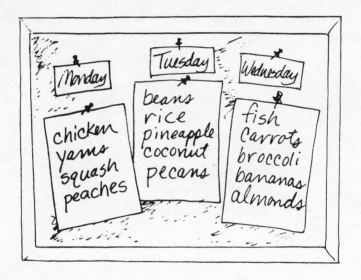

A rotated diet is a varied diet (and a carefully planned one too). In following such a diet, you eat different foods every day and try not to repeat a food more often than every four to seven days.

Rotating your diet isn't easy. Yet, if you and your family are loaded with allergies, a rotated, diversified diet will help you identify foods that bother you now and prevent other hidden food allergies from developing in the future.

ROTATED DIETS

FOOD	DAY 1	DAY 2	DAY 3	DAY 4
Meats	Beef	Chicken	Shrimp	Trout
Fruits	Orange	Banana	Pineapple	Apple
Vegetables	White potato	Sweet Potato	Carrot	Squash
Grains	Wheat	Amaranth	Rice	Buckwheat
Nuts	Pecan	Almond	Cashew	Filbert
Fats & Oils	Butter	Safflower oil	Walnut oil	Sunflower oil
Miscellaneous	Milk	Egg	Chocolate	Carob

The Chemical Problem

Chemical Contaminants in Your Food*

Let's suppose you follow the instructions in this book and you improve. Yet, you continue to experience symptoms. And such symptoms are caused by something you're eating.

In this situation, you'll have to search further. And you may find you are bothered by sensitivity to the chemicals in foods and in food containers (including cans, plastic wrappings and boxes). Many chemical contaminants in foods are derived from petro-chemicals and coal tars. Others come from antibiotics and insecticides.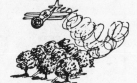

Here are examples:

Bananas picked green are usually exposed to a petroleum-derived gas, ethylene. So are apples, pears, oranges and tomatoes.

Chickens may contain antibiotics, hormones and other chemicals.

Sugar is usually treated with chemicals of various sorts during processing.

Peelings on fresh fruits and vegetables often contain insecticide and herbicide residues. They also may be coated with mineral oils and waxes to give them an attractive shine.

French fried potatoes may be treated with chemicals to prevent discoloration.

Beef and pork may contain chemicals and hormones of various sorts. Some are administered to the animal before slaughtering; some are added to the meat as preservatives.

---

*Adapted from material prepared by Dr. Theron Randolph.

Tap water often contains chemicals from a variety of sources. These include insecticides or weed killers which remain in the water in spite of purification and filtration; chemicals added to the water including fluorine and chlorine; chemicals picked up from plastic pipes or copper pipes; industrial residues and nitrite fertilizers which seep into the water table.

Tracking down a hidden chemical allergy is even more difficult than tracking down hidden food allergy. However, it can be done. Here are suggestions that may help you.

1. Use well, spring or distilled water in glass bottles. (Water in plastic bottles will be chemically contaminated.)
2. Obtain foods from organic sources. (Some farmers, growers and packers specialize in raising and producing foods which are as free of chemical contamination as humanly possible. You'll find a list of some of them in the Food Sources section.)
3. Use no canned or packaged food in diets to determine chemical sensitivity.
4. If you use commercial foods, purchase those in glass containers. (Avoid canned foods and those wrapped in plastic.)

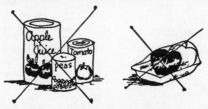

5. Use glass jars or containers (rather than plastic) to store foods in your own refrigerator.
6. Purchase meats, fruits, vegetables, grains from growers in your area who use organic farming methods. (You can obtain such a list of growers by writing to PREVENTION MAGAZINE, 33 E. Minor St., Emmaus, Pennsylvania 18049.)

7. Foods less apt to be chemically contaminated include:

Fish and Meat

Seafood and meat from which the fat has been stripped prior to cooking.

Vegetables

Potato (undyed and home-peeled), turnips, egg plant, tomato (if field ripened), carrots (but not bagged in plastic), squash, okra, green peas and green beans.

Fruit

Organically grown fruits.*

Miscellaneous

Nuts (in shell only), Brazil nuts, coconut, walnut, hickory nut, pecan, filbert, hazel nut.

Sweetening agents

Honey, maple and sorghum.

Fats and Oils

Olive, cottonseed, peanut, sesame, soy, safflower, sunflower, walnut and linseed oils.

---

*Such fruits may be hard to find. Yet, you're probably aware that in 1987, chemically-contaminated watermelons from California made a lot of people sick. Also, strawberries, apples, pineapples and other fruits may be chemically contaminated by insecticides. Or they may be treated by other chemicals to retard spoiling.

More on The Chemical Contaminants in Your Food—and What You Can Do About Them

In their book, *An Alternative Approach to Allergies,* Theron G. Randolph, M.D. and Ralph Moss, Ph.D., tell of a man who develops "searing attacks of head pain" after eating apples. Dr. Randolph said, "I naturally diagnosed him as allergic to apples."

Subsequently, the man gathered apples from trees in an abandoned orchard which hadn't been sprayed in years. And surprisingly, he was able to eat the apples with complete abandon. He developed no headache or other adverse reactions.

In following up on this clinical observation, Randolph noted that *many patients who reacted to fruit (and other foods) weren't reacting to the food, but to the chemical pollutants in or on the food.*

It is now becoming obvious to many observers that many of our foods are contaminated. These contaminants include:

- Chlorinated hydrocarbons in meats which enter the animals' bodies by way of feeds.

- Insecticides and insecticide residues.

- Herbicides (weed killers) and fungicides.

- Other toxic substances which are added to or sprayed on foods to prevent deterioration or to improve their appearance.

- Lead and other chemicals from automobile exhausts which contaminate vegetables, fruits or grains from fields adjacent to heavily traveled roads.
- Aflatoxin, a powerful carcinogen produced naturally by a mold that grows on crops including field corn and peanuts.
- Antibiotics (which are added to 60% to 80% of beef, poultry and swine feed).
- Bacteria and parasites.

Tetracycline (for animal use)

Chemical contamination of our food seems to be increasing. It's a subject you should know more about. The best current source of information: *Americans for Safe Food,* 1501 16th Street, NW, Washington, DC 20036, (202) 332-9110. This coalition, spearheaded by the Center for Science in the Public Interest (CSPI), is a non-profit organization advocating progressive public health policies.

Here are excerpts from a 50-page booklet, *Guess What's Coming to Dinner,* published by ASF in March, 1987.

GUESS WHAT'S COMING TO DINNER

Contaminants in Our Food

Americans for Safe Food

CSPI CENTER FOR SCIENCE IN THE PUBLIC INTEREST

"Our food is contaminated. From pesticide residues on fruits, vegetables and grains to antibiotic-resistant strains of Salmonella bacteria in our meat, to traces of powerful animal drugs in poultry, invisible chemicals and germs permeate our food supply. You won't see these dangerous residues on any ingredient list . . . the law doesn't require it.

"Consumers feel betrayed having learned about the dietary causes of heart disease, cancer, stroke and diabetes, millions of Americans have begun eating more fish and poultry, whole grains, fresh produce and low-fat dairy products. All too often, however, these otherwise wholesome foods are tainted, and government regulation amounts to little more than a false promise of protection.

"Chemicals also poison our environment. They contaminate ground waters, rivers and lakes; kill wildlife; and trigger the spread of bugs and weeds that are resistant to pesticides.

"Once consumers learn abut the dangers associated with so many of our foods, the next step is to press for safe alternatives. A growing demand for safe food will eventually cause brokers and farmers to make changes . . . changes that will be to everyone's advantage in the long run, with the possible exception of the chemical and drug manufacturers. That is the goal of *Americans for Safe Food,* and the shelves of some supermarkets bear evidence that the process has already begun.

"The campaign is a positive one . . . (its) goal is realistic . . . crops and animals can be grown with far fewer chemicals than they are today. Furthermore, *Americans for Safe Food* is not calling for an immediate end to the production of chemically-treated food. It is simply demanding what many consumers are demanding: A safe alternative."

Here are a few of the suggestions in the booklet under the heading, WHAT YOU CAN DO:

1. Organize an *Americans for Safe Food* coalition in your community (write to ASF to find out how).
2. Visit the managers of your local supermarkets. Urge them to offer more contaminant-free foods.
3. Get informed, then organize a local "Safe Food Day" community forum, or public debate on contaminants in food.
4. Prepare a list of local sources of contaminant-free food.
5. Write, and tell your friends to write, letters to the editor of your local newspaper. The shorter your letters are, the more likely they are to be published.

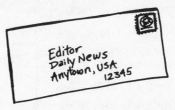

Whether you're troubled by food sensitivity reactions or whether you aren't, I urge you to send $5 to *Americans for Safe Food.* They'll send you a copy of *Guess What's Coming to Dinner* and additional information.

Now here's still another suggestion: Raise some of your own food. Or find a farmer's market which features produce which has been grown "organically." Such food has been fertilized with

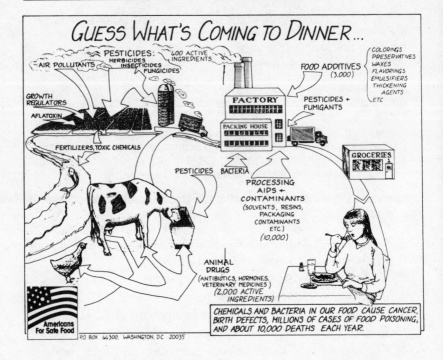

GUESS WHAT'S COMING TO DINNER...

CHEMICALS AND BACTERIA IN OUR FOOD CAUSE CANCER, BIRTH DEFECTS, MILLIONS OF CASES OF FOOD POISONING, AND ABOUT 10,000 DEATHS EACH YEAR.

natural compost (a fertilizing mixture composed of manure, peat, leaf mold, lime, food scraps, etc., mingled and decomposed).

To learn more about organically-grown foods, join Natural Food Associates (NFA), a non-profit educational organization, P.O. Box 210, Atlanta, Texas 75551. Your $15 membership fee will include a one-year subscription to *Natural Food and Farming*, the official journal of this organization.

Here are titles of typical articles in recent issues of this interesting publication:

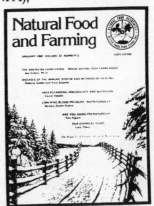

Sick Soil, Basic Cause of Poor Health
Food Irradiation—Another Reason to Buy Natural Foods
Quinoa (pronounced Keen'wa)—the Super High Protein
  Cereal of the Inca Empire
Our Chemical Feast
Lower Blood Pressure—Nutritionally
Bugs, Weeds and Free Advice

Advertisements in this journal provide information about organically grown grains, flours, fruits, nuts, beef and chicken.

Here's more. Just as this book was going to press, I received a copy of the May 1988 issue of AMERICAN HEALTH, with a picture of Robert Redford on the cover. Also featured on the cover were a series of articles in a section entitled, CLEAN UP TIME: FIGHTING OR OUR ENVIRONMENT. These articles told about Robert Redford's fight for a cleaner environment, pesticides in strawberries, a mother's fight for clean water and how and why to plant a garden.

Here are excerpts from an article, TAMING THE KILLER STRAWBERRIES.

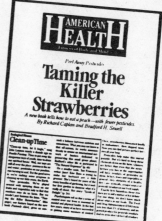

"Once, strawberries blossomed briefly in mid summer, then skipped town. Now, you can find picture perfect berries all year long.

"Pesticides help make this marvel possible. But, it's hard to keep these chemicals down on the farm: Chances are better than even that the strawberries you buy in the supermarket will have residues of pesticides on them. In fact, fruits and vegetables in general—key elements of a healthy diet—are, ironically, a major source of pesticide residues in our food supply."

One of the AMERICAN HEALTH authors suggests writing to Americans for Safe Food (ASF). He also recommends the book, PESTICIDE ALERT, which is available from bookstores. It can also be ordered from the National Resources Defense Council (send $6.95 plus $1.55 shipping) to NRDC, Publications Department, 122 East 42nd Street, New York, NY 10168.

Recipes

Introduction

All of the recipes in this section have been prepared, served and enjoyed by my long-time colleague and associate, Nell Sellers and by Marge Jones, R.N.* Each of these experienced professionals has developed an interest in allergen-free cooking because of their own multiple sensitivities.

You can obtain additional information about food allergy including suggestions and recipes for allergy cooking in Marge's publications:

MASTERING FOOD ALLERGIES—a monthly newsletter
THE ALLERGY SELF-HELP COOKBOOK (Rodale Press)
ALLERGY RECIPES, BAKING WITH AMARANTH (a booklet)

For more information, write Marge Jones, MAST ENTERPRISES, 2615 North Fourth Street, Suite 677, Coeur d' Alene, Id. 83814.

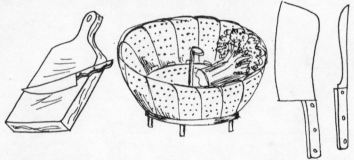

In discussing recipes for elimination diets for her newsletter, Mastering Food Allergies, Marge Jones commented, *"The best recipes are no recipes at all."*

I agree. In carrying out your elimination diet, feature simple, unprocessed foods including vegetables, fruits, meats, rice, barley, oats, and unprocessed nuts from a health food store (or nuts in shell).

Shop around the perimeters of your supermarket rather than going up and down the aisles looking for foods you can eat. Here's why: With a few exceptions, most packaged, processed and

---

*Marge is co-authoring (with me) THE YEAST CONNECTION COOKBOOK, Professional Books, publication date—early 1989.

canned foods contain hidden ingredients including sugar, corn syrup, yeast, soy and other substances which would mess up your diet.

Purchase some of your foods from a farmer's market or a health food store which features chemically uncontaminated fresh foods.* Although chemically-free foods are hard to find, informed consumers all over the country are demanding and obtaining better and safer foods—even from the major food processors and chain stores.**

Prepare foods simply. Broil, bake and boil them. Make sure your cooking utensils are "antiseptically clean" and free of traces of foods that could interfere with the accuracy of your diet trials.

Here now are a few recipes you can use for Elimination Diet A. You may also be able to use several of them for "the long haul." However, if you find that you're allergic to only one, two or three foods, as for example, milk and wheat or eggs, yeast and corn, consult one of the food allergy cookbooks in the reading list. Such books will help you prepare interesting meals which avoid the dietary ingredients you're sensitive to.

Cole Slaw

shredded cabbage
grated carrots
minced green pepper or pineapple
Cashew No-Egg mayonnaise

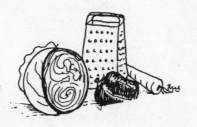

---

*See also pages 91–95.

**For more information, send a stamped, self-addressed envelope to Americans For Safe Food, 1501 Sixteenth Street N.W., Washington, DC 20036.

Chicken-Rice Soup

6 cups chicken stock (water in which chicken has been stewed)
½ cup brown rice (raw)
⅓ cup chopped onion
⅓ cup sliced or shredded carrots
⅓ cup celery, thinly sliced
1 tablespoon oil (olive, walnut or canola)
1 cup cooked chicken, diced
salt
2 tablespoons chopped parsley

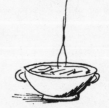

Heat chicken stock to boiling. Add rice and simmer 35 minutes.

Sauté onion, carrots, and celery in oil for 5 minutes and add to soup. Add chicken, correct seasoning and just before serving, add parsley. Yield: Approximately 6 servings.

Waldorf Salad

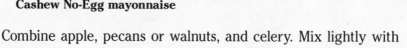

1 apple, cored and chopped
celery chopped
1 tablespoon chopped pecans or walnuts
Cashew No-Egg mayonnaise

Combine apple, pecans or walnuts, and celery. Mix lightly with mayonnaise until all pieces are coated. Chill.

Cashew No-Egg Mayo

An adaptation of old-fashioned boiled dressing—basically seasoned, thickened nutmilk.

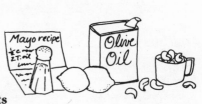

½ cup raw cashews or other nuts
¾ cup water
1–2 tablespoons lemon juice, or ¼ to ³/₈ teaspoon corn-free
vitamin C crystals (derived from sago palm)
2 tablespoons oil
1 tablespoon arrowroot or kuzu starch
½ teaspoon dry mustard
¼ teaspoon salt, or to taste
dash cayenne, optional (go easy for youngsters)

Grind the nuts to a fine powder in a blender. Add the water and blend 1 minute. Add the lemon juice, oil, starch, mustard, salt and cayenne.

Blend until very smooth, stopping twice to scrape the bottom. Pour into a saucepan. Stirring or whisking constantly over medium heat, bring to a boil and simmer 2 or 3 minutes until it's thick.

Allow to cool 10 minutes, then stir in lemon juice or the vitamin C crystals, and correct the seasonings to your taste.

Transfer to a glass jar and store up to 2 weeks in the refrigerator. If you wish, top your salad with a few cashews or whatever nuts you made the dressing with.

Marge Jones, R.N.

Almond or Cashew Butter and Banana Salad

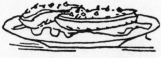

Slice a banana into fourths. Coat with a layer of soft nut butter. Sprinkle chopped almonds, cashews or pecans over the top. Serve on a lettuce leaf.

Chicken Salad

cooked chicken, diced
celery, chopped
salt and pepper to taste
Cashew No-Egg Mayonnaise

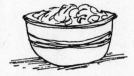

Oat Bran Muffins

These rise well, are good for you (if you can have oats) and taste great. I developed the carrot version for those who need to limit fruits.

⅔ **cup rolled oats**
2 **teaspoons baking soda**
½ **teaspoon salt**
1½ **cups oat bran**
1 **cup mashed ripe banana or applesauce or puréed carrots (add**
    2–3 tablespoons water to sliced cooked carrots; purée to get
    applesauce consistency)
¾ **cup pineapple or apple juice**
¼ **cup oil**
2 **eggs, separated**

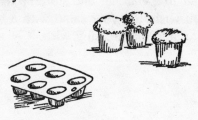

Optional Additions:

½ **teaspoon nutmeg**
⅓ **cup chopped nuts**
4 **tablespoons currants**

Grind rolled oats into flour in a blender. Add the soda, salt, and nutmeg, blending to mix well.

Pour dry ingredients into a small bowl and stir in the currants or nuts, if you want them. Measure the oat bran into a larger bowl.

Without washing blender, put the mashed banana, juice, oil and egg yolks in it. Blend for 60 seconds and pour over the oat bran. Stir to moisten, then allow to soak for 10 minutes.

Preheat the oven to 400° and prepare the muffin tins with paper cups or oil. Beat egg whites in a small bowl until they hold a soft peak.

Add dry ingredients to the oat bran mixture and stir only to wet the flour. Quickly fold egg whites in with a rubber spatula. Divide into 12 muffin cups and pop in the oven at once. Bake 15 minutes or until lightly brown and crusty. Serve with Pineapple "Jam."

Marge Jones, R.N.

Pineapple "Jam"

Strain crushed pineapple in its own juice, any size can.
Reserve the juice and put the fruit in a blender. Purée
until smooth or leave it a bit chunky; serve warm or cold.
If you prefer a thinner consistency add a little of the re-
served juice.

When it's thick, it's a jam, and thinner, it's a topping or sauce.
You can use fresh, sweet pineapple or fresh frozen instead of
canned.

Marge Jones, R.N.

Baked Sweet Potatoes

3 or 4 medium-sized sweet potatoes
1 or 2 tablespoons oil

Scrub sweet potatoes with a brush under running water, until
thoroughly clean. Dry on paper towels, then rub a little oil over
the outer surface until potatoes are lightly oiled all over.

Place potatoes in a baking pan or iron skillet and bake in a 350°
oven for about 1 hour or until tender when pierced by a fork.

Special Meat Loaf

2 pounds ground beef
⅓ cup Minute Tapioca
⅓ cup onion, finely chopped
1½ teaspoon salt
¼ teaspoon pepper
1 medium tomato, chopped

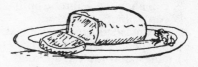

Combine all ingredients, mixing well. Pack into a 9" x 5" x 3" loaf
pan. Bake in a 350° oven for 1 to 1¼ hours. Unmold on serving
platter and slice as needed. May be served hot or cold. Actually
slices better cold. If you have leftovers use for brown bag lunches
with rice crackers or serve for at-home lunch with hot buttered
brown rice or Spanish rice and a salad.

Oven Baked Chicken

8–10 pieces chicken
1 cup permitted flour (amaranth, buck-
wheat, oat, arrowroot, etc.)
1 teaspoon salt
¼ teaspoon pepper
½ teaspoon paprika
1 tablespoon walnut or safflower oil

Skin the chicken pieces and rinse well.

Mix flour and seasoning in a paper bag. Add 2 or 3 pieces of chicken at a time and shake to coat. Continue until all the chicken is coated.

Place the chicken in a single-layer in a 9″ x 13″ pan. Dribble a little oil from a teaspoon onto each piece of chicken. Bake in a 350° oven for about 1 hour or until chicken is tender. Serves 5–6.

Buckwheat Banana Bread

Grinding your own unroasted groats adds about 7 minutes.

2 tablespoons flax seeds
½ cup water
1¼ – 2 tablespoons "white" (unroasted)
buckwheat groats, whole
½ cup pumpkin seeds
½ teaspoon salt
3 teaspoons baking powder
½ cup chopped walnuts, optional
¼ cup walnut or other oil
2 cups mashed, ripe banana (about 5 bananas)
¼ teaspoon vitamin C crystals (sago palm)
1 tablespoon vanilla, optional

Preheat oven to 375°; oil 8 x 4″ loaf pan.

Combine flax seeds and water in small saucepan, bring to full boil, then turn off heat; allow to soak until needed.

In blender, grind buckwheat ½ cup at a time. Place a strainer over mixing bowl and pour the ground flour into it. Rub through with a spoon. Return any unground chunks to blender with the next batch of groats. Repeat grinding until 1¼ cups have been processed. Put a tablespoon of flour into oiled pan and tap to cover bottom. Invert pan over mixing bowl and tap excess back into flour.

In blender combine pumpkin seeds, remaining 2 tablespoons buckwheat groats, salt and baking powder (plus any spice you choose to add) and grind together until it's a fine meal, stopping machine to scrape bottom once or twice. Add seed mixture to flour, add chopped walnuts, if you want them, and mix well.

(Be sure you have a mark on blender for 2¼ cups; if not, measure that much water into blender jar, mark and discard water.)

Measure oil into blender. Break banana into 1 inch chunks and liquify. Add one banana at a time, turning machine off to measure. Stop adding bananas at 2¼ cups. Add vitamin C crystals and vanilla. Mix.

Pour liquid mixture over flour. Using a rubber spatula, stir with a few swift strokes to moisten evenly but don't beat hard. Quickly scrape batter into a pan and pop into oven. Bake 45–50 minutes, til brown and toothpick test is dry. Remove pan to wire rack to "sweat" for 10 minutes, then turn out on rack to cool completely before slicing.

Serving Suggestions: Mash a ripe banana and whip lightly with a fork until it's the consistency of whipped cream. Lay 2 slices of the Buckwheat Banana Bread on a plate and top with Banana Creme Topping. This "Banana Shortcake" = whole breakfast!

Marge Jones, R.N.

Flat Bread/Chapatis/Tortillas

Tested successfully with these flours: buckwheat, chick-pea, oat, rice, rye, barley, amaranth and quinoa.

1 cup of any flour and extra to roll in
½ cup water, approximately
Pinch of salt, optional

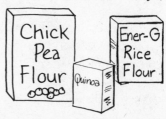

Stir together a few minutes until ball forms. Add extra flour or water, if needed for "play dough" consistency. Break off golf-ball sized pieces of dough, flatten and roll thin (about 6 inches across) on well-floured board. Pre-heat griddle.

If breads are well-floured, they bake on a dry griddle, with no oil added. They take only a few minutes on each side to bake.

Variations: Add about 2 teaspoons oil to rice flour, which is quite dry. OK to add to others, too, but not necessary. May also add a little cinnamon or nutmeg.

Note: For sandwiches, open-faced work best. Try a nut butter topped with sliced fruit for breakfast or lunch. Some flat breads can be rolled, others are too crisp.

Experiment. They're fun and so easy.

Marge Jones, R.N.

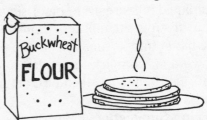

Buckwheat Pancakes

1 cup buckwheat flour
pinch of salt, optional
1 cup water, about

Combine ingredients using enough water to make medium-thin batter. Let it stand for a few minutes then bake on a hot griddle.

These flour and water pancakes are simple to make and work well for sandwiches, as well as for breakfast. Their texture is firm and a little dry.

For variation, replace up to ⅓ of the flour with ground nuts or seeds, or add one tablespoon of oil and/or ¼ teaspoon of cinnamon. The ingredients you choose depend on your own limitations. Serves 2.

Note: All commercial buckwheat flours I've ever seen are from roasted groats and have a strong flavor. If buckwheat is new to you buy whole, unroasted groats and grind in your blender for a mild pleasant taste.

Marge Jones, R.N.

Amaranth Pancakes/Flatbread

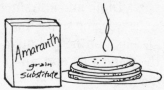

½ cup Amaranth flour
dash of salt
¼ teaspoon baking soda
½ cup water
4 teaspoons oil
¹/₈ teaspoon vitamin C crystals (from sago palm, not corn)

Combine all but the C crystals. Allow to stand a few minutes (or refrigerate overnight). Preheat a griddle until a drop of water will "dance" on it. Stir in C crystals quickly, adding a little more water if needed to make a medium-thin batter.

Drop 1 or 2 tablespoons on a hot griddle to make 4 or 6 inch pancakes. Cook until they appear dry around the edges, turn and bake the other side. These require a bit more time on each side than wheat pancakes do.

Serve with any fruit topping or nut or seed butter, or make your favorite sandwiches. Or omit the soda and C crystals, for a slightly heavier texture; but still delicious!

Keep them thin so they cook in the middle. Oil your griddle lightly.

Try this: Add a dash of cinnamon to the batter and serve with apple butter sweetened with apple juice. Eat them out of hand as you would toast. If the cakes were already cooked and are frozen, pop them in a toaster oven to warm briefly or toast them crisp, if you'd rather. If you've no toaster oven arrange the pancakes on a wire rack on a cookie sheet and warm for 5 to 10 minutes in a standard oven.

Marge Jones, R.N.

Quinoa Pancakes/Flatbread

½ cup quinoa, uncooked
½ cup of water
pinch of salt, optional

Measure quinoa into a pan, add cold water and swish well with your hand. Drain into a strainer, return wet quinoa to the pan and repeat the washing step a few times until the water remains pretty clear. Drain. Put the wet quinoa in a blender (invert the strainer over the blender jar and tap it). Add all but about 2 tablespoons of the water, and salt.

Grind on low speed. Stop to scrape the sides as needed. Finish by blending a minute on high. Pour the batter into a small bowl. Add remaining water to the blender jar and blend briefly to rinse. Pour liquid into the batter and stir in. Allow it to stand a few minutes (or refrigerate overnight).

Spoon onto a hot griddle, spreading them out with the back of the spoon. Bake on a hot griddle, as above. Lightly oil the griddle before starting to bake.

Serve with fruit or nut butter for breakfast, or make wonderful sandwiches for lunch.

Marge Jones, R.N.

Popsicles

Puréed watermelon, honeydew or cantaloupe make great popsicles—just pour into a special mold or ice cube tray. When partially frozen stick cocktail toothpicks or wooden sticks in the center of each.

Apple Crisp

(Developed by Marge Jones for *The Yeast Connection Cookbook*)

1 or 2 very ripe pears (1 cup purée)
1 tablespoon lemon juice
3 tablespoons walnut oil
¾ cup rolled oats
½ cup oat bran or oat flour
½ cup chopped walnuts
1 teaspoon cinnamon
dash of nutmeg, freshly ground
¼ teaspoon salt, optional
1½ tablespoons Minute Tapioca
5 cups sliced apples (golden delicious work especially well)

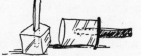

Core, peel and dice the pears. Purée them together with vitamin C crystals or lemon juice in a blender. In a small bowl mix ⅓ cup of the purée with the oil, rolled oats, oat bran or flour, walnuts, spices and salt. Set aside.

In a large bowl, combine and mix well ⅔ cup of purée and the Minute Tapioca.

Peel and slice apples, adding them to the tapioca-pear mixture as they're ready. Toss apple slices to coat, and pour into an oiled casserole or 8x8″ glass baking pan. Distribute the crumbs evenly on top. Cover with lid and bake at 350° for 30 minutes. Remove the lid and continue to bake 10–15 minutes until bubbly and apples are tender. Cool a little before serving.

Marge Jones, R.N.

Oat Biscuits

(Developed by Marge Jones for *The Yeast Connection Cookbook*)

2⅓ cups rolled oats
½ teaspoon baking soda
¼ teaspoon salt
¼ cup canola oil
⅓ cup puréed fresh pear, ripe and sweet
1 tablespoon lemon juice

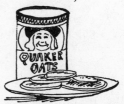

In a blender, grind 2 cups of rolled oats into flour. Measure 1 cup of flour into a small bowl and add the soda and salt. Mix well.

In a medium bowl whisk the oil, puréed pear and lemon juice together. Stir in the flour mixture and beat hard 10–12 strokes. Add more flour, 2 tablespoons at a time, until dough forms a soft ball.

Scatter the remaining flour on a board or waxed paper, and turn half of the dough onto the board. Turn it over, patting the dough into a smooth ball, to coat it with flour on all sides. Pat it into a thick, flat patty. Scatter the remaining rolled oats (not ground) in two large circles on a cookie sheet.

Lay the first dough in the middle of a circle of rolled oats, on the cookie sheet, and repeat the procedure with the other half of the dough. Now roll or pat both circles of dough to 6 or 7 inches across and ½ inch thick. Gather any loose rolled oats from the cookie sheet and sprinkle the tops with them, patting them in slightly. Cut each into 8 wedges. Makes 16 delicious biscuits. Keep well for 3 to 4 days.

Variation: To make these a bit like a cookie, put chopped nuts into the top surface.

Marge Jones, R.N.

Oatmeal Cookies

Not a great "Keeper"—Very good when fresh, but they go downhill in a few days. (Adapted by Marge Jones for the *Yeast Connection Cookbook*)

3 cups rolled oats
1 cup oat flour
½ teaspoon salt
1 teaspoon baking soda
½ teaspoon cinnamon, optional
1½ cups mashed banana
½ cup oil
⅓ cup chopped nuts or seeds, optional

Preheat oven to 350°. Mix the dry ingredients. Mix oil and bananas. Stir the two together and add nuts or seeds if you want them. Drop by teaspoons on oiled pan or cookie sheet. Bake at 350° for 16 minutes.

Makes about 3 dozen cookies.

Nickie Dumke, Denver CO, submitted by Ann Fisk

Delicious Sweet Potatoes

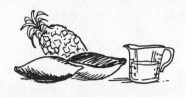

3 or 4 medium sweet potatoes
⅛ to ¼ cup fresh pineapple
1 to 2 ounces water

Scrub and peel potatoes and cut in half lengthwise. Arrange them in a baking dish. Mix the pineapple and water in your blender and pour over the potatoes. Bake at 400° for 45 to 60 minutes, depending on the size.

Marge Jones, R.N.

Descriptions of Hidden Food Allergies—and Other Adverse Food Reactions—in the Medical and Lay Literature

The References from the medical literature cited in this section are listed alphabetically in the reference section, pages 213–221.

INTRODUCTION

For the Physician and Other Professionals: Chances are, you'll be surprised—just as I was—when you see how many allergists (and other physicians) have described food-related problems in the medical literature. Included are people from many branches of medicine including both practitioners and academicians.

Yet, non-IgE mediated food sensitivities have—in general—been ignored by most physicians in "the medical mainstream." The status food allergy has occupied during the past several decades reminds me of an address delivered by one of my favorite medical school professors, the late Oscar Swineford, M.D. of the University of Virginia.

In 1964, this distinguished American allergist called allergy "the bastard of medical education."* At that time, most allergists felt that they were "second class citizens" in the eyes of their colleagues, especially those in university centers.

Then, following the discovery of immunoglobulin E (IgE) later in the 1960s (plus other advances), the field of allergy and immunology gained credibility and respectability.

Speaking before a group of science writers in Baltimore in 1970, Dr. Richard S. Farr of the National Jewish Hospital and Research Center in Denver, said in effect, "We've now identified four major types of immune reaction:

"Type I Immune Reaction. This type of reaction is mediated through a fraction of the blood called 'gamma E reagin' or IgE. Positive Type 1 reactions are seen following skin tests to pollens, molds, animals danders, dust and less commonly, with food.

---

*Swineford, O.: Journal of Medical Education, October 1964.

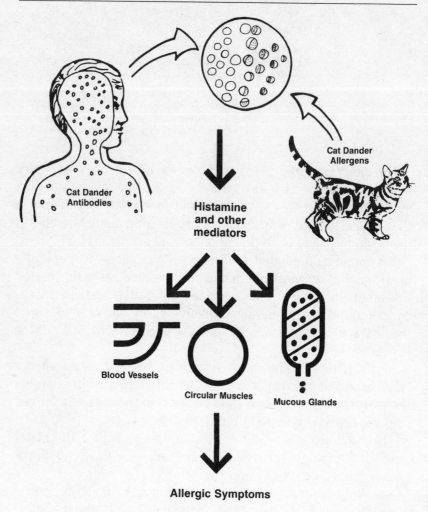

Cat Dander Antibodies

Cat Dander Allergens

Histamine and other mediators

Blood Vessels

Circular Muscles

Mucous Glands

Allergic Symptoms

"Type II Immune Reaction. Although this type of reaction cannot be detected by skin tests, it can be identified by other sophisticated laboratory procedures.

"Type III Immune Reaction. In this sort of reaction, the skin test becomes positive in about 12 hours and reaches a peak in 24 to 48 hours.

"Type IV Immune Reaction. Reactions of this type are delayed. A positive skin test will not turn red until 18 to 24 hours and will not reach a peak until 72 hours."

According to Dr. Farr, to make a diagnosis of allergy, you must explain it on the basis of one of these known immunologic mechanisms. "This is a very stringent definition," said Dr. Farr, "because it *insists* that an immunologic mechanism be identified as causing or contributing to the cause of illness."

Yet, concurrently and even before, *a handful of leaders in the field of allergy and immunology, talked and wrote about adverse food reactions which could not be explained on an immunologic basis.* In addition, countless other observers, including both physicians and non-physicians, described these adverse food reactions.

On the pages that follow, you'll find a surprising number of references to food sensitivity. I found them fascinating and hope that you will, too.

For Non-Professionals: Even though this section is designed especially for professionals, it should interest you. You'll read about "typical allergic symptoms" (sneezing, wheezing, cough and sinus) which are food related. You'll also see that many physicians have noted that food sensitivities can cause headache, fatigue, irritability, nervousness, musculoskeletal discomfort, urinary problems and other disorders.

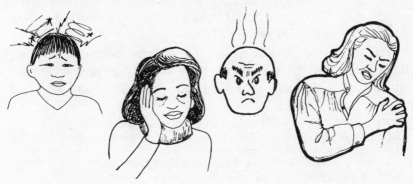

In spite of these observations and reports, (as you may have found out) the role of food sensitivity in causing such symptoms has—until recently—been ignored. When usual laboratory and other tests haven't proved an explanation, these symptoms have usually been blamed on "hypochondriasis" or "neurosis."

EARLY DESCRIPTIONS OF FOOD RELATED PROBLEMS

Over 2,000 years ago, Lucretius said, "One man's meat is another man's poison." And Hippocrates noted, "There are certain persons who cannot readily change their diet with impunity; if they make any alteration in it for one day, or even for a part of a day, are greatly injured thereby. Such persons, provided they take dinner when it is not their wont, immediately become heavy and inactive, both in body and mind . . ."*

And in the first chapter of Daniel in the Old Testament you can read about the successful use of an elimination diet.**

Daniel and three of his friends were being trained to serve in Nebuchadnezzar's royal court and they were required to consume the same food and wine as other members of the court. But Daniel and his friends didn't want to partake of the royal fare.

So Daniel went to his supervisor and said, "Test us for ten days. Give us vegetables to eat and water to drink. Then compare our appearance with that of the young men who are eating the food of the royal court and base your decision on how we look."

The supervisor agreed to let them try the special diet for ten days. When the time was up, the three young men on the elimination diet looked healthier and stronger than all of those who had

---

*Hippocrates, On Ancient Medicine (Adams, 1886) as quoted by Iris R. Bell, M.D., Ph.D., Clinical Ecology, A New Medical Approach to Environmental Illness. Common Knowledge Press, Bolinis, CA, 1982, p. 7.

**Daniel 1:20, Good News Bible: The Bible in Today's English Version (New York): American Bible Society, 1976, pp. 954–955.

been eating the royal food. So from then on, they were allowed to eat vegetables instead of what the king provided.

"At the end of the three years set by the king . . . they became members of the king's court. No matter what questions the king asked or what problems he raised, these four knew ten times more than any fortune teller or magician in his whole kingdom."

During the next 2,000 years, adverse food reactions were occasionally mentioned in the lay literature. However, not until the twentieth century were such reactions referred to in the medical literature.

DESCRIPTIONS OF HIDDEN FOOD ALLERGIES IN THE MEDICAL LITERATURE DURING THE TWENTIETH CENTURY

During the First Three Decades: In a fascinating two-volume book, THE FOOD FACTOR IN DISEASE (published in 1905) Dr. Francis Hare discussed the food/mood relationship. He described patients with a variety of disorders who were relieved when they eliminated common food from their diets.

In the introduction to his book, Dr. Hare tells how he "stumbled on" the relationship of diet to migraine headaches, a disorder that was generally thought, at that time, to be a primary—usually hereditary—disorder of the brain.

Dr. Hare then told of similar dramatic results in another patient who had been placed on a special diet and he noted, "The attacks of migraines ceased absolutely from the day on which he commenced dietetic treatment: They returned within a fortnight after the cessation of treatment. They continued to recur there forward with the old regularity . . . Such results appear inexplicable, except on the hypothesis that migraine, in these cases at least, was a food disease."

In his continuing discussion, Dr. Hare also noted that he found "on searching through Hyde Salter's classic work, ON ASTHMA, numerous instances of the salutary influence" of dietary changes in helping patients with asthma.

In discussing the role of diet and mental illness, he referred to a patient report by George Keith:

"A man had been in an asylum for the greater part of his life. From time to time he refused food, and it was put into his stomach by a tube. At last his health quite failed, so much that it was considered useless to force hunger any longer upon him. He was left to die in piece. He did not die and more than that, he recovered his sanity and was able soon to leave the asylum."

Dr. Hare also said,

"I've heard of a lunatic who escaped from his asylum and wandered about several days without food, recovering his sanity before he was found."

He told of another patient,

"An elderly gentleman came to me complaining of intense mental depression, recurring daily between the hours of 10 a.m. and noon . . . His breakfast consisted of porridge and milk with sugar, followed by eggs and bacon, or a chop of steak, also bread, butter and marmalade. The more depressed he became, the bigger the breakfast he ate in order to 'keep his strength up':

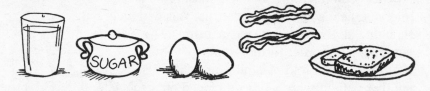

"As a result, his depression intensified further. He was ordered a lighter . . . breakfast. Porridge, sugar and bread were interdicted . . . The depression ceased concurrently with the alteration of diet and has not returned."

Since the book by Hare, numerous physicians during the 20th century described systemic and nervous system reactions caused by allergies, including food allergies. Here are some of these reports:

In an article in the AMERICAN JOURNAL OF DISEASES OF

CHILDREN, published in 1916, B. R. Hoobler noted nervous system disturbances in allergic infants and young children. He commented upon "their restlessness, fretfulness and sleeplessness"

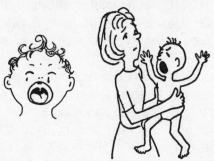

and their tendency to irritability. Then in 1923, W. R. Shannon, a Minnesota pediatrician, reported seven patients with generalized symptoms due to allergy. He especially emphasized the involvement of the nervous system.

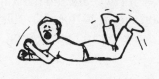

The same year, May reported a case of a 19 year-old girl who had recurrent attacks of extreme drowsiness which could be precipitated by eating a food she was sensitive to. And Duke called attention to the occurrence of fatigue and other generalized symptoms in allergic patients. In his experience, the symptoms were usually caused by foods.

During the 1930s, 40s and 50s: Beginning in 1930, the prolific pioneer food allergist, Albert Rowe, Sr., of Oakland, California, described respiratory, digestive, nervous and other symptoms in many of his patients with food allergies. The nervous symptoms included drowsiness, irritability, fatigue, weakness, and slowness of thought. Other patients, especially children, showed irritability

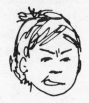

and incorrigibility. Rowe used the term "food toxemia" to apply to these patients with systemic manifestations which were food related.

In the 1940s H. J. Rinkel began to publish similar observations on patients with delayed-onset food sensitivities. He used the term *"masked food allergies"* to describe the reactions in these patients.

Like other medical pioneers, Rinkel "stumbled" on the relationship of food sensitivity to generalized body symptoms. Here's the Rinkel story as told by Theron Randolph:

Rinkel, a poor boy, was attending medical school during the great depression in the 1930s. His family were egg farmers and they sent him crates of eggs every month to help maintain his nutrition.

Rinkel's general health was good. Yet, he was troubled by a severe allergic rhinitis of undetermined cause. According to Dr. Randolph, streams of mucus would pour from the young medical student's nose at all times.

At some point, Rinkel decided to experiment with his diet. And when he avoided eggs for 4 to 5 days *his nose stopped running. Then after eating a piece of egg-containing angel food cake, he fell to the floor unconscious!*

Following this experience, Rinkel came up with the following hypothesis: a person with a *"masked"* (hidden) allergy to a food he eats regularly may show persistent symptoms including rhinitis, headache, fatigue and muscle aches. Yet, the relationship of the symptoms to common foods is rarely recognized.

But, if the person avoids a food causing these symptoms for a four to twelve day period and then eats the food again, an obvious, even violent reaction may occur.

The Rinkel observations have influenced countless physicians during the past forty years and the Rinkel method for carrying out an elimination diet is featured in this book. To detect a *masked, hidden* or *delayed-onset food allergy,* the following steps must be carried out:

1. A symptom diary must be maintained while the person is on a regular diet.
2. Suspected foods must then be eliminated for four to twelve days.
3. During the period of elimination, if the symptoms are food related, they should improve substantially or go away.
4. The symptoms should return in a decisive, even exaggerated manner when the foods are eaten again.

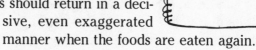

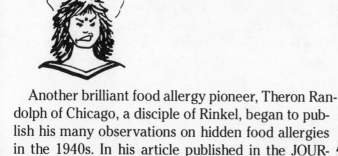

Another brilliant food allergy pioneer, Theron Randolph of Chicago, a disciple of Rinkel, began to publish his many observations on hidden food allergies in the 1940s. In his article published in the JOURNAL OF PEDIATRICS in 1947, Randolph described for the first time the facial pallor, eyelid edema and allergic shiners often seen in children with allergies.

In 1951, Rinkel, Randolph and Michael Zeller collaborated in a classic book *FOOD ALLERGY. This book describes, in detail, the clinical picture, the concepts, the diagnosis and management of delayed-onset food allergies and outlines, for the first time, the rotating diversified diet.

Another pioneer of this period, Arthur Coca, of New York, a person with severe food sensitivities, published a book on the subject in 1942, FAMILIAL NON-REAGINIC FOOD ALLERGY. In this book, Coca emphasized the great frequency of unsuspected food

---

*This book, originally published by Charles C. Thomas, Springfield, IL, was republished by the New England Foundation for Allergic and Environmental Diseases. It is available from Dickey Enterprises, 635 Gregory Rd., Fort Collins, CO 80524.

allergies. He also noted that methods other than skin tests were needed to make a diagnosis. Coca utilized changes in the pulse rate after a test feeding to determine these hidden food allergies. However, because his observations were considered "controversial," they were rejected by most of his peers at that time and later.

Concurrent with the observations of Rowe, Rinkel and Randolph and Coca, other reports appeared in the medical literature describing systemic and nervous system reactions due to both foods and inhalants. Yet, because they were scattered in the literature of different specialities, few physicians were aware of them.

In 1954, another food allergy pioneer, Frederic Speer of Kansas City published the first of his reports on what he termed *"the allergic-tension-fatigue syndrome."* Here are excerpts from one of his articles:

"Patients who suffer from motor fatigue complain of weakness, fatigability and achiness . . . Many of these patients find it difficult to carry on sustained activity of any kind that require more than the normal amount of physical and mental rest."

Speer also noted the frequency of aching in the shoulders, arms, legs, neck and other muscles in allergic patients. He also described the sensory fatigue which occurs in the food sensitive patient:

"The patient describes himself as tired, weary, droopy, sluggish, apathetic, exhausted, torpid, sleepy, listless, languid and dull . . . A striking feature of allergic fatigue first noted by Randolph is that it is usually not relieved by rest. Prolonged sleep may, in fact, make it considerably worse."

In 1959, James Breneman (of Galesburg, Michigan), reported the first sixty-five cases of food allergy producing nocturnal enuresis in children. And in 1965, he reported his findings on another hundred patients with similar problems. Like Rowe, Rinkel, Randolph and Speer, Breneman noted the relationship of food allergy to recurrent abdominal pain, malaise and other systemic and nervous system manifestations in his patients. In the Preface of his recent book, he commented,

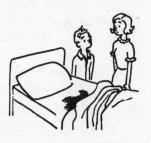

"In 1959, I was first impressed with the importance of food allergy and illnesses, not always considered as allergic diseases . . . Food allergy has replaced syphilis, as the great imitator. Food allergy and sensitivity mimic symptoms of almost any disease . . . *Any patient with confusing symptoms, prolonged complaints, poor treatment response . . . might recover amazingly on a week of diagnostic elimination diet. It's harmless and can be astonishingly effective.*"

During the 1960s, 70s and 80s: In 1961, I described food-related, systemic and nervous system symptoms in fifty of my pediatric patients. (See also *A Special Message to the Physician,* pages 13–21.) All these patients complained of fatigue and appeared pale with dark circles or shadows under their eyes. With one exception, all were troubled by nasal congestion and nervous system symptoms (irritability, restlessness, inability to concentrate, anxiety, tearfulness, peevishness and perversity). Over half complained of headache and abdominal pain. Still others were troubled by muscle aching and symptoms in other parts of the body.

In the ensuing years, in my office practice of pediatrics and allergy, I saw thousands of patients (including both adults and children) whose chronic symptoms improved or disappeared after they identified food troublemakers and changed their diets. I reported my findings in various professional journals.

Rowe, Rinkel, Randolph and Speer continued to write about hidden food allergies.* Moreover, their teachings influenced their students, associates and hundreds of other physicians. Yet, most physicians (including allergists) paid little attention to hidden or delayed-onset food allergies.

Interest in the systemic and nervous system manifestations of food allergy began to accelerate in the 1970s. Leaders in the field of allergy and immunology who described such symptoms included William C. Deamer, Oscar Lee Frick (and associates), Frederick Speer and John W. Gerrard.

In an award-winning presentation, delivered before the section on allergy on the American Academy of Pediatrics, October 20, 1970, Deamer commented on the deceptive nature of food allergy and the resultant difficulties in diagnosing and treating it.

Deamer noted the unreliability of food skin tests and the value of elimination trial diets in studying patients with fatigue, irritability, headache, abdominal pain, musculoskeletal discomfort, pallor and respiratory tract symptoms. In his discussion, he commented,

"Ascribing the asthma and allergic rhinitis which may be relieved by the omission of certain foods (and brought on by their reintroduction), to allergy disturb some purists. They point out the frequent absence of a demonstrable antibody and the need for better evidence that allergy is involved at all. Many would be happier with the term "food intolerance." They are even more reluctant to accept the concept of the allergic tension-fatigue syndrome.

*Rinkel died in 1963, Rowe died in 1973 and Speer died in 1986. Randolph, now in his 80s, continues to write, lecture and care for patients.

"There can be no doubt, however, of the role specific foods may have in causing these symptoms nor of the fact that the respiratory tract symptoms they produce appear to be, in every way, identical to those caused by accepted antigens."

"It is probable that every pediatrician and physician in general practice sees such cases . . . I cannot help but feel that all physicians caring for children would do well to become acquainted with the allergic tension-fatigue syndrome with the frequency with which foods . . . are responsible for it."

At the same meeting of the American Academy of Pediatrics, Bill Deamer and Lee Frick presented a scientific exhibit entitled, *The Allergic Tension-Fatigue Syndrome*. This exhibit featured a large color picture of a typical child with food allergy—pallor, allergic shiners, mouth breathing and an overbite. These typical allergic facies were also recognized, photographed and publicized by Meyer B. Marks of the University of Miami in a monograph published by the Upjohn Pharmaceutical Company. Marks also reported his observations in the medical literature on numerous occasions.

In spite of the observations by Deamer, Speer and others, the *Allergic Tension-Fatigue Syndrome* wasn't accepted as a valid diagnosis by many physicians. For example, in a 1970 article, physicians from another university medical center presented an entirely different point of view.

In this article, *Recurrent Abdominal Pain in Childhood*, R. T. Stone, M.D. and G. J. Barbero, M.D., described their findings on 104 children with recurrent abdominal pain. And they blamed the pain and associated symptoms (headache, limb pain, bedwetting, dizziness and pallor) on a functional basis and made a diagnosis of "irritable bowel syndrome."

A number of physicians responded to Stone and Barbero article. James P. Kemp, M.D., Assistant Clinical Professor of Pediatrics (Allergy) and Co-Director of the Pediatric Allergy Clinic and Training Program (University of California, San Diego) was among those who expressed a different point of view. Dr. Kemp noted that the authors of the article were unaware of the article in PEDIATRICS, *Systemic Manifestations Due to Allergy*. Or if they were aware of it, they chose to disregard it. And Dr. Kemp commented,

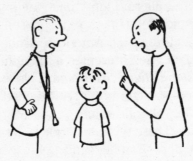

"The use of such a wastebasket diagnosis as the "irritable bowel syndrome" offers the patient little relief other than knowing that 101 other individuals suffer, perhaps needlessly, from the same condition. Although none of these children may have food allergy, I've seen many patients who, with similar symptoms, have improved by following the hypo-allergenic diets and whose symptoms have recurred once specific foods were returned to the diet . . .

"The authors, resistance to treat by dietary manipulations . . . is a terrible oversight at the very least. Because allergy patients do have these symptoms, I cannot disregard them and hope that they will just go away . . . What is not looked for, certainly in many cases, will not be found."

Other physicians who disagreed with the Stone and Barbero conclusions included Joseph D. Bullock, M.D., William C. Deamer, M.D., Oscar L. Frick, M.D., Ph.D., James R. Crisp, III, M.D., Stanley P. Galant, M.D. and William H. Ziering, M.D. (Department of Pediatrics, Pediatric Allergy Division, University of California Medical School, San Francisco) who commented,

"We should like to draw attention to another organic diagnostic possibility for at least some of the cases (of recurrent abdominal pain). The *tension-fatigue syndrome* (TFS) is a symptom complex occurring mainly in children but also in adults. The TFS is usually due to food allergy. It manifests itself in many different ways in many systems. There's a striking similarity of symptoms manifested by these 102 children and children with the TFS.

"Any one of the components of the TFS may be the patient's chief complaint. We've seen patients with this syndrome who were investigated for a brain tumor because of headaches or studied for anemia because of pallor and fatigue. Others have undergone extensive bowel studies because of abdominal pain or have been diagnosed as 'rheumatic' because of leg aches and fever. One patient had a muscle biopsy because of leg pain and fatigability.

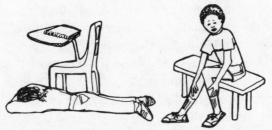

"Two patients were referred to a psychiatrist because of their behavior . . . We do not suggest that all, or even the majority, of these patients have food allergy. We feel that some of them, however, fulfill many of the features of the *tension-fatigue syndrome.*"

In spite of the comments by Deamer, Kemp and others indicating that children with recurrent abdominal pain, headache and limb pains could be relieved by an elimination diet, two subsequent articles in PEDIATRICS blamed such symptoms on psychological causes.

One of these articles, *School Phobia—The Great Imitator: A Pediatrician's Point of View*, was written by Barton Schmitt of Denver. A similar article was written by Jacob Oster entitled,

Recurrent Abdominal Pain, Headache, and Limb Pains in Children and Adolescents. Again, Bill Deamer responded:

"In one series of 96 children with the allergic tension-fatigue syndrome seen in our pediatric allergy clinic and privately, the six most common complaints . . . other than respiratory tract symptoms . . . were in order: Headache, 61%; Recurrent abdominal pain, 58%; Nervous tension, 52%; Pallor, 52%; Fatigue or tiredness, 47%; Limb pain, 36%.

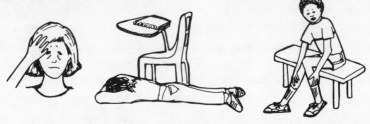

". . . *all patients were . . . successfully treated for the stated symptoms by elimination of specific food allergens . . .* In most instances, either a sibling or a parent had a history of similar symptoms attributable to food sensitivity."

Douglas H. Sandberg, M.D. of the University of Miami also responded. Here are his comments:

"The article by Dr. Jacob Oster describes very well the symptoms of the complex which is now recognized by allergists under the name, the *allergic tension-fatigue syndrome.* As a pediatrician working primarily with gastrointestinal disorders, I have come in intimate contact with many children and parents with this symptom complex. In many of them I have seen remarkable improvement or complete disappearance of such symptoms with institution of elimination diets, restricting common food allergens such as milk, wheat and corn.

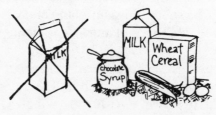

"These children usually show the characteristic pallor, circles under their eyes . . . In addition, they're often found to have a poor pattern of linear growth. I'm writing to add my voice as a non-allergist to those who would like to see the *allergic tension-fatigue syndrome* recognized as a valid diagnosis."

J. Rainer Poley, M.D. and Mira Bhatia, M.D. of the Children's Memorial Hospital, University of Oklahoma Health Science Center commented, "We agree wholeheartedly with the comments made by Drs. Deamer and Sandberg . . . In our experience, the most frequent offending proteins are milk proteins, soy proteins . . . as well as corn and the citrus family."

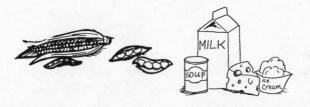

Bill Deamer continued to write and teach his students and fellows about delayed-in-onset food allergies until his death in 1983. Here's another example published in the February, 1973 issue of CURRENT MEDICAL DIGEST:

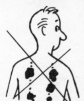

Food allergy occurs much more often than is generally appreciated and is often overlooked. One reason for this is that only one type of food allergy, the prompt, onset type (such as is often due to shell fish, peanuts, etc.) has a reasonably good correlation with positive skin tests.

In the other, the delayed-onset type, skin tests as well as other immunologic tests are useless . . . "Onset" refers to the time lapse between ingestion of a food and resultant symptoms, which is often a matter of hours or even days.

Recognition of delayed-onset food allergy is further compli-
cated by the fact that the symptoms it causes are rather ordinary
and non-specific. They're more apt to suggest a number of other
causes—and allergy is rarely thought of as likely.

Because immunologic tests cannot be relied upon, recognition
of delayed-onset food allergy depends on skillful history taking.
One must search diligently and seek out the following signs and
symptoms:

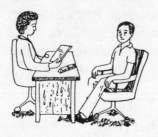

Headache, fatigue, nervous tension, pallor,
musculoskeletal aching . . . and respiratory
tract symptoms such as nasal congestion,
coughing or wheezing.

Together with recurrent abdominal pain, these
symptoms make up the syndrome of delayed-onset
food allergy. This is often referred to as the *allergic
tension-fatigue syndrome.*

Here are descriptions of food-related problems by a distinguished American physician, Walter C. Alvarez, who retired from
the Mayo Clinic at the age of 65 and who continued to write for
physicians and the public until he retired again at the age of 90.

In the foreword to the book, ALLERGY OF THE NERVOUS SYS-
TEM, edited by Frederic Speer, Dr. Alvarez commented,

"Back around 1930, I was one of the small group of men who
were studying food allergy and had learned that it can produce a
dull brain. For years before I knew I was highly sensitive to
chicken, I suffered from what I call 'dumb Mondays,' when I was
too dull to do much constructive work like writing. Finally I discovered that the bad Mondays were due to the Alvarez family's habit

of eating chicken for Sunday dinner. When I stopped eating chicken, that was the end of my troubles on Monday.

"Then one day, when I happened to tell my dear friend, Dr. Clifford Sweet, an able pediatrician about my dumb Mondays, he said, 'That gives me an idea; among my not young patients, I have many with 'dumb Monday'; I must inquire now to see if they have what you had.'

"A month later, when I saw Cliff, he told me that a study had soon shown that the dumb Monday children were suffering from food allergy, and it came most often on Mondays because on Sunday the child usually ate something not eaten during the rest of the week.

"Cliff said, 'I now have a big 'dumb Monday' club.'"

John Gerrard, Professor of Pediatrics, Emeritus, University of Saskatchewan, in a delightful 77-page book, UNDERSTANDING ALLERGIES (published in 1973) told of patients he'd seen whose bedwetting ceased promptly when the patient stopped drinking milk. He also noted that symptoms of other sorts including nasal congestion, drowsiness, irritability and hyperactivity were also related to unsuspected foods.

Dr. Gerrard described reactions of Tim who had been placed on a restricted diet for two weeks and then given a glass of milk to drink and in an hour a second glass.

"Tim promptly became a *ball of fire.* He went wild and was quite uncontrollable." In commenting on this child and other similar patients, Dr. Gerrard said,

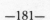

"At first I found it hard to believe that harmless foods could so change a child's personality; but many parents have made confirmatory, unsolicited observations, and I'm now fully convinced that in ways we do not yet understand, the allergic child's, and adult's too, behavior can be altered and modified as dramatically by foods as it can be altered by drugs.

"The following examples indicate the bizarre nature of these problems. A medical student . . . has to avoid foods containing corn because corn makes him feel so drowsy that he can hardly keep his eyes open. An internist has found that he has to avoid foods containing egg and wheat because these two foods make him irritable and irascible . . . Two pediatric acquaintances both find that coffee which keeps most people awake puts them to sleep."

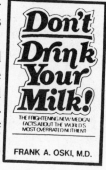

Here's further support for the role of foods—especially milk—in causing systemic and nervous system symptoms in both adults and children.

Frank A. Oski, M.D., a former Professor and Chairman of the Department of Pediatrics at the State University of New York (Upstate Medical Center), now is Professor and Chairman of the Department of Pediatrics at Johns Hopkins School of Medicine. In a 1977 book, co-authored by John D. Bell, Dr. Oski commented:

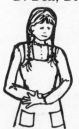

"Most people, including physicians, believe that allergies to foods . . . produce only such classical symptoms as skin rashes, respiratory symptoms or gastrointestinal disorders. There is a growing body of evidence, however, to suggest that certain allergies may manifest themselves primarily as changes in personality, emotions, or in one's general sense of well-being . . .

"The child or adult with motor fatigue always seems to feel weak and tired . . . Excessive drowsiness and torpor are typical.

These children are particularly listless in the morning. They are difficult to awaken and appear never to have had a good night's sleep.

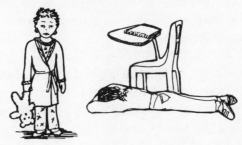

"Tension is the other major manifestation of food allergy. These children will appear restless and in a constant state of activity. They fidget, grimace, twist, turn, jump and just never seem to sit still. Many of these children are also excessively irritable and can never be pleased.

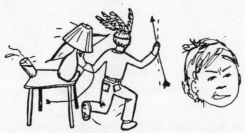

"Although the *tension-fatigue syndrome* is the most common manifestation of food allergy, it is by no means the only one. Vague recurrent abdominal pains, repeated headaches, aching muscles and joints and even bedwetting have been observed as symptoms of food allergy . . .

"*Although I've emphasized the role played by food allergies in producing symptoms in children, adults appear equally prone to the problems produced by foods . . . The food* most responsible for the symptoms in both adults and children is whole cow milk."

Doris Rapp, M.D., a Magna Cum Laude graduate of the University of Buffalo, a Fellow of the American Academy of Allergy and a Clinical Associate Professor of Pediatrics at the State University of New York at Buffalo, had been engaged in "traditional" allergy practice for eighteen years.

Then, in 1975, for the first time, she became interested in hidden or delayed-in-onset food allergies. In the last thirteen years, she has conducted medical research, published medical articles, has lectured, made videotapes and movies and has written books* for the public and for professionals about her observations on hidden or delayed-onset food allergies.

Here's a brief summary of Dr. Rapp's observations on the correct way to carry out an elimination diet. In a letter to the editor published in PEDIATRICS (Volume 67:937, 1981), she emphasized the following points:

1. If a child is sensitive to several foods, eliminating only one of them may not help.
2. In challenging a child who has improved on an elimination diet, the amount of the food required to trigger a reaction may vary because children are individuals.
3. If you stop eating a food you're sensitive to for several weeks, you may be able to eat it again without difficulty for a while before the symptoms return.
4. To determine whether a food is producing symptoms, it should be eaten again after it's been avoided for five to twelve days.
5. A food may not cause a reaction when it's eaten again if it hasn't been avoided in all forms.

In a report in CLINI-PEARLS (a continuing medical education publication for the practicing pediatrician), editor Walter Tunnessen, Jr., M.D., State University of New York, Upstate Medical Cen-

---

* Dr. Rapp's most recent Book *The Impossible Child* is available From P.A.R.F., P.O. Box 60, Buffalo, NY 14223-0060.

ter, Syracuse, New York 13210, told of an eight-year-old boy who comes into the pediatrician's office with lethargy and dark circles under his eyes but with an essentially normal examination except for a few shotty cervical lymph glands. In commenting on this patient, Dr. Tunnessen said,

"Maybe the problem does have an emotional basis. But before we label this child as such, consider the great masquerader—food allergy. This just happens to be a favorite diagnosis of mine . . . I cannot prove it with esoteric or even routine laboratory tests. *The proof of the pudding, so to speak, is in some simple dietary elimination . . . a benign procedure, most often painless, requiring no hospitization and downright inexpensive.*

"The culprits I find most common are milk, chocolate and eggs, although cane sugar, corn and wheat should also be considered. Removing these foods from the diet, a few at a time for a week or two, is all that is necessary. Should a child improve, the eliminated foods are reintroduced. If symptoms recur, the foods are again eliminated.

". . . The manifestations of food allergy are legion. Motor symptoms may include overactivity, restlessness and clumsiness; sensory tension may be reflected in irritability, insomnia or hypersensitivity to pain or noise. Fatigue symptoms include tiredness, achiness and the like . . . pallor, circles and nasal stuffiness are almost invariably present. Headache, abdominal pain, enuresis, increased sweating and salivation and infraorbital edema are commonly present . . .

"I . . . had been a doubting Thomas until my son responded to dietary elimination . . . Do we need hard data in the form of laboratory confirmation to support every diagnosis? I think not. 'Soft data,' subjective signs and symptoms can be applied just as rigorously to reinforce our hypotheses."

In a 1980 report, Sandberg, McLeod and Strauss discussed the relationship of food hypersensitivity to kidney disease. Here are excerpts from this report:

"Recently, evidence for food hypersensitivity has been reported by Matsumura and associates. This sensitivity does not appear to be IgE mediated, although it may occur in atopic individuals."

Sandberg also discussed the relationship of food allergy to albumin in the urine. He pointed out that Matsumura and his colleagues have demonstrated that food sensitivity may be a significant factor in causing benign protein in the urine and in causing nephrosis. He commented,

"Postural proteinuria is often associated with symptoms related to other organ symptoms, i.e., fatigue, gastrointestinal complaints, etc., which occur commonly in children with food sensitivities. *Detection of food sensitivity in their patients was accomplished by history, food diaries, elimination diets and subsequent trials of suspected foods* . . . In 136 patients, Matsumura found 72 instances in which food produced postural proteinuria."

In order of frequency, milk was the cause in 30 patients, eggs in 20 instances, soybean in 17 instances and pork, red beans and tuna in a few individuals. Disappearance of postural proteinuria was demonstrated when the specific foods were eliminated from the diet."

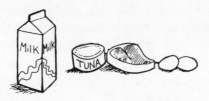

Sandberg then discussed the relationship of food sensitivity to membranous glomerulopathy, anaphylactoid purpura nephritis and minimal change nephrosis. In his summary he commented,

"There is an appreciable evidence implicating hypersensitivity reactions in pathogenesis of certain types of renal disease. The data presented above strongly suggests that sensitivity to food may be an important component to the multi-factorial etiology of renal disease in such patients."

Still further support for the role of allergies to foods can be found in the 1980 book, ALLERGIES TO MILK, by Sami L. Bahna, Professor of Pediatrics, Cleveland Clinic Foundation and Douglas C. Heiner, Professor of Pediatrics at the University of California (Torrance).

Although this book was devoted mainly to IgE mediated milk allergies, it also discussed the *allergic tension-fatigue syndrome* and other manifestations of delayed-in-onset food hypersensitivities.

In discussing the *allergic tension-fatigue syndrome,* the authors said,

"The onset is often insidious and symptoms may go unrecognized for years, with frequent visits to physicians, multiple investigational procedures and ineffective medications. The diagnosis is often missed, both because of the subjectivity of symptoms and because of the lack of a reliable laboratory test . . .

". . . *We have occasionally seen typical cases with a dramatic response to the correct elimination diet.* A poor response is often noted in patients with multiple allergens where the recognition and elimination of offending agents is often incomplete . . . Undoubtedly, many of the symptoms reflect a chronic hypersensitivity state, perhaps related to excessive release of chemical mediators, or lymphokines into the circulation."

These authors also commented on the urinary manifestations in people with allergy and they cited the observations of Matsumura, Gerrard and Breneman, and in referring to Breneman's findings, they said,

"In 1959, Breneman described 24 cases of enuresis in which cow's milk, alone, or in association with other foods, was suspected to be a causative allergen. In all patients, the enuresis disappeared after an elimination diet was begun. From his experience, Breneman believed that food allergy was a common cause of nocturnal enuresis with cow's milk being the leading causative allergen."

In a discussion entitled, *Food Problems,* in the October 1981 issue of CUTIS, Steven G. Tolber* commented,

"I would like to address those reactions which occur many hours, even days (following the ingestion of a food), and are not associated with positive skin tests."

Tolber then described a 35-year-old man who had "frequent migraine-type headaches for a period of three years. Finally, he went to see an allergist. At that point, it was discovered that chocolate and corn were related to the headaches. Skin tests to these foods, as well as to a standard screening panel, were completely negative . . . I was extremely interested in this case. As you might guess, I was the patient."

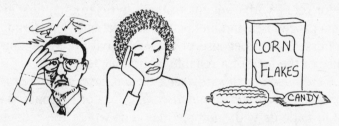

In his continuing discussion, Tolber briefly reviews the controversy which exists among allergists when food-related problems are discussed. Some believe in them enthusiastically and fanatically while others deny their existence. In referring to the skeptics, he said,

"I think it is unfair for these physicians to throw away all observations made by many excellent clinicians although they remain unexplained . . . The fact that there is not complete scientific evidence to back up an observation does not necessarily invalidate that observation.

". . . Food avoidance can be tried for a short specific period of time to see if there's an improvement. I also think it is important to challenge the patient to each of the suspected foods individually to see if there's any worsening of symptoms . . .

---

*Private Practice of Allergy and Clinical Immunology, Clinical Assistant Professor of Pediatrics, University of New Mexico College of Medicine, Albuquerque, NM.

This whole area seems so sensitive to some clinicians that they completely ignore and disbelieve what the patient tells them with regard to foods. I believe that this prejudice is completely unscientific and is not in the best interest of the patient . . . This is not an easy field, but it certainly is not impossible. But why take my word for it? Go and observe."

In a commentary published in the January 1982 issue of the JOURNAL OF THE ARKANSAS STATE MEDICAL SOCIETY, Harold Hedges of Little Rock commented,

"The longer I practice medicine, the more I am convinced that many illness are caused by what we eat, drink or breathe. I have practiced medicine since 1963 as a partner in Little Rock General Practice Clinic. I have treated many patients with obvious diseases—diseases which can be seen by the naked eye or obviated by sophisticated lab and x-ray examinations . . .

"I've also treated many patients with diseases and disorders which I could neither see with the naked eye nor specifically obviate by the same examinations. I have labeled (in good faith) these many problems as:

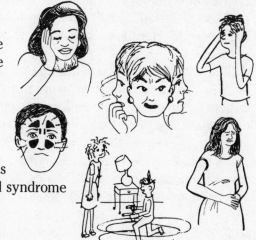

1. Tension headache
2. Fatigue syndrome
3. Chronic sinusitis
4. Irritable colon
5. Depression
6. Nerves
7. Anxiety
8. Situation reactions
9. Hyperactive child syndrome
10. Hypochondriasis
11. Nervous stomach

Some I even laid on the poor lowly virus (I thank God for viruses)—even if I couldn't prove it so, the patient couldn't prove me wrong!"

Dr. Hedges then goes on to tell how he learned to help many and perhaps most such patients using four to seven day elimination diets and identifying the food troublemakers by adding food back, one at a time. In his continuing comments he said,

"I would suggest that each of you reading this be a 'doubting Thomas' and don't believe any of this until seeing it work. Try it on some of your most difficult and puzzling cases, cases which you've already had the usual customary workup for that particular complaint . . .

"It certainly is not the panacea for all chronic complaints, but there are enough successes to make the extra time worthwhile. *The numbers who respond to this approach will surprise you as it has me . . . Look for the chronic patient whose symptoms you clear. You will be heaped with thankfulness."*

Robert M. Stroud a former member of the Editorial Board of the Journal of Allergy and Clinical Immunology, reported on a multi-center study of 45 patients with arthritis. Special attention was paid to the possible role of foods in causing arthritis. All patients were fasted initially and then foods were reintroduced. Here are excerpts from Dr. Stroud's report:

"The average duration of fasting was 6.6 days with a range of 4 to 9. No major complications were noted . . . During the fast the patients characteristically had increasing discomfort for 2–4 days . . . There was a statistically significant improvement in joint swelling, grip strength (and other objective tests).

"In a majority of patients, the changes were dramatic . . . On the average for each patient, 17.2 foods were non-reactive; 7.5 of the reactive foods were classified mild to moderate; and 2.8 were major to severe . . . *Fruit and vegetables demonstrated a statistically lesser reactivity than cereals and animal protein* (page 52)."

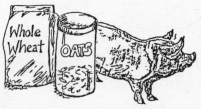

In his award-winning Bela Schick lecture for 1984 entitled *Deciding the Future for the Practice of Allergy and Immunology,* William T. Kniker commented on what he terms "the very narrow scope of clinical disease" dealt with by most allergists and immunologists. Yet he continued,

"There are countless . . . millions . . . of individuals who have unrecognized adverse reactions to various antigens, foods, chemicals and environmental or occupational triggers . . . The acquired disease may be limited to body surfaces or may involve a puzzling array of organ systems causing the patient to visit a number of different specialists who are unsuccessful in recognizing that an allergic or adverse reaction is going on."

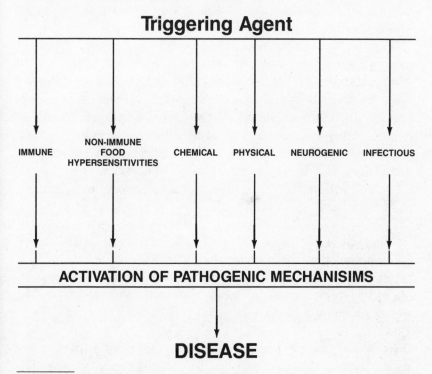

Chart adapted from Kniker, W. T., "Deciding the Future for the Practice of Allergy and Immunology," *Annals of Allergy,* 55:110, 1985.

In a subsequent presentation at the annual meeting of the American College of Allergists, Phoenix, Arizona, January 1986, Dr. Kniker again emphasized the importance of adverse food reactions in causing symptoms in allergic patients. And he said in effect,

"Probably the bulk of clinically relevant food reactions are delayed . . . As far as the pathogenic mechanisms, a lot of study needs to be done. But already it's clear that virtually every cellular system involved in inflammation . . . has been shown to be activated in one or more of these reactions . . . In the delayed group, not only can you see classic allergic reactions, but a very variable presentation involving a variety of organ systems, either singularly or in combination . . .

"Diagnostically, the immediate reactions are easy. The patient usually figures them out and never sees a doctor. If they do, all you do is confirm what the patient already knows. Your skin tests and your RAST tests and your challenges . . . merely make it clear that . . . when they eat so and so, they get sick within an hour. But in case of delayed reactions . . . , the history . . . is of limited help . . . Diagnostic tools, short of diet and manipulation are very unsatisfactory. *But in most cases, elimination and challenge . . . and . . . dietary manipulation will lead to a reasonable management* . . . Let's look at some data.

"Recently, Ortolani in a study in Milan, Italy of 210 adults found that the chronic rhinitis in 25% of his patients was largely triggered by something they ate, 13% were caused by foods and another 11% were caused by additives."

In his continuing discussion, Kniker described other studies which showed that food sensitivities contributed to asthma. The range in papers he cited varied from 10% to 68%. Although Kniker noted that a lot of these studies are flawed, he said,

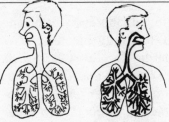

"It is indisputable that food ingestion caused asthma in many of these cases."

In the remainder of his discussion, Dr. Kniker urged the hundreds of allergists in the audience to become interested in food allergies and he said,

"The practice of allergy and immunology is potentially the greatest in medicine. It transcends all specialities, all diseases . . . We are the specialists in the community concerned with adverse reactions to a variety of things we drink, eat, breathe, touch and smell."

He pointed out that allergists need to do a lot more than study and treat their patients with skin tests and shots and that they need to be aware that allergies can cause symptoms in parts of the body other than the respiratory tract and the skin.

In his continuing discussion he pointed out that food-related symptoms have long been recognized in infancy. Yet, he said that food sensitivities were also common in older children and in adults.

"I guarantee you when you look into the foods, all of a sudden you'll find that rhinitis or the asthma or whatever, can come under control in a good many of those cases because you've discovered the missing triggers . . . Stomach pains, constipation, diarrhea, myalgia, arthralgia, irritability, poor sleeping habits, enuresis and other symptoms seen in children, at times, are also food related.

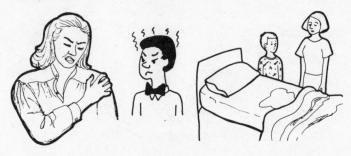

"What about laboratory or diagnostic tests . . . The skin tests or the RAST test only means you're sensitized. It doesn't mean you're allergic . . . *Every one of these tests, skin tests, RAST or ELISA . . . have an unacceptably high rate of false positives and false negatives. Other tests . . . are still under investigation . . . Measurement of antibodies of other sorts, IgG subclasses, IgA to foods, IgG; immune complexes, (etc.) . . . But any of these either are not at all proved yet or are so expensive or cumbersome that they're not practical.*"

In the concluding portions of his address, *Dr. Kniker pointed out that in studying and helping these patients, it comes down to diet manipulation.*

And in a workshop presentation on food allergy at the 44th Annual Conference of the American College of Allergists, in Boston in November 1987 Dr. Kniker said,

"Doctors, I think we need to change our thinking. Just remember that food sensitivities cause trouble and the day will come when we will look at our patients and say, 'How much of our patients' problems are caused by inhalants and how much caused by foods . . . rather than just looking at one or the other."

Food Allergies, Food Hypersensitivities and Elimination Diets Come Into the Medical Mainstream

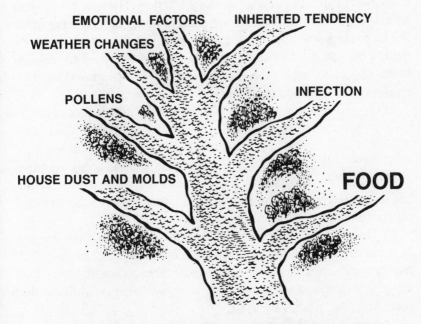

Allergies and Hypersensitivities

Early in 1987, a comprehensive new book appeared on the medical scene. Its title: FOOD ALLERGY AND INTOLERANCE. Eighty-three physicians and other scientists contributed to this book. Here are comments from the Preface:

"As all who deal in the field will know, food allergy is an exciting, challenging, exasperating and sometimes controversial subject. Its study should be a clinical science with diagnosis based on a combination of clinical observations and scientific investigations . . .

"The field of food allergy has generally been considered to be a clinical art rather than a laboratory science. There is more than an element of truth in this since clinical observations have often not been supported by reliable diagnostic tests or even laboratory data. This has led to skepticism of some of the clinical associations, especially when the mechanisms of any proposed food allergies are not understood . . .

"There has been a strong tendency for the conventional physician to say that if the mechanism is not understood then food allergy does not exist . . . This is, of course, unacceptable . . .

". . . To make a diagnosis (of food allergy) certainly requires clinical skill but does not necessarily need a complete understanding of the mechanisms underlying the disease process or an exact understanding of the etiology . . .

"A thread running through (this book) . . . is that *the cornerstone of diagnosis of food intolerance is the removal of that food from the patient's diet with concomitant improvement (or not) of the patient's symptoms and their reappearance on adding that food back* . . . (italics by WGC)

"We hope that the emphasis placed in this book on the correct methods for the diagnosis of food allergy may result in fewer patients being classified as food allergic without good evidence; but in contrast we hope, too, that increased understanding of food allergy will make physicians more aware that at least some of their polysymptomatic patients may have an organic basis for their complaints."

The entire issue of the November 27, 1987 issue of the JOURNAL OF THE AMERICAN MEDICAL ASSOCIATION consisted of a Primer on Allergic and Immunologic Diseases. It was prepared by the American Academy of Allergy and Immunology and edited by Richard F. Lockey, M.D. and Samuel C. Bukanz of the University of South Florida College of Medicine, Tampa, Florida.

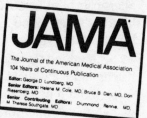

Chapter six of this Primer by Hugh A. Sampson, M.D., Rebecca Hatcher Buckley, M.D., and Dean D. Metcalf, M.D., dealt with food allergy. In describing the clinical features of food allergy, these authors discussed immunologically mediated reaction to foods which they point out are "expressed clinically by diversity of signs and symptoms, ranging from abdominal pain to generalized anaphylaxis."

They also noted that "in addition to the GI system, food allergy also can be expressed in extraintestinal target tissues, particularly the skin and, less frequently, the respiratory tract."

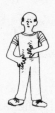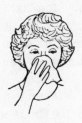

Yet, they seemed to express skepticism over the relationship of food allergy to systemic and nervous system symptoms described by many other physicians and they said, "Behavioral disturbances and depression as manifestations of food allergy have never been demonstrated conclusively."

In discussing diagnostic techniques they emphasized the importance of a careful his-

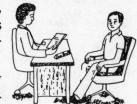

tory. They also suggested the use of skin tests and radio-allergosorbent tests (RAST) and the use of double-blind or single-blind, placebo-controlled oral challenge with suspected foods. Yet, they also recommended the use of elimination diets. And in discussing such diets, these physicians stated,

"Although much more tedious than in hospital, placebo controlled oral challenges, this approach has been used as an outpatient diagnostic aid for many years. *The principle is somewhat the same, i.e., if the offending food is removed from the diet of the affected individual, the food-induced illness will resolve . . .*

> My Symptoms
> Fatigue
> foggy feeling
> stuffy nose
> headache
> stomach pain
> muscle aches

". . . It is useful for the patient to remain on his or her usual diet for approximately 10 to 14 days before any special diet is initiated. During that time, the patient should record the type and amounts of foods ingested and the occurrence and character of adverse reactions. This record is useful in searching for suspected foods and establishing baseline symptoms against which the success or failure of elimination diets may be measured . . .*

. . . "Initiation of a severely limited diet is warranted if the removal of one or several foods from the diet is not successful, in eliminating symptoms or if multiple food sensitivities are suspected . . .

. . . "*Caution* must be taken to instruct the patient to take nothing by mouth but the foods on the diet and water. Oral medications including aspirin, vitamins and laxatives must be avoided when possible. Continuation of symptoms fol-

---

*In the diet instructions provided for in TRACKING DOWN HIDDEN FOOD ALLERGIES, I recommend only a diary of three days before beginning the elimination diet. Yet, whenever feasible, I agree that a longer period of time for establishing base line symptoms can be even more helpful.

In their concluding remarks, these authors commented,

"To diagnose food allergy, it is first necessary to exclude the possibility that one of a number of other causes might be responsible for the signs and symptoms."

lowing restricted diets indicate that symptoms are not due to foods or other avoided substances.

"The unlikely possibility of the individual foods on the restricted diets are causing symptoms may be eliminated by substituting other foods known not to correlate with symptoms. However, if symptoms resolve on the restricted diet, resumption of a normal diet should be accompanied by a return of symptoms and subsequent resumption of the restricted diet should alleviate these symptoms."

In their continuing remarks they emphasized the importance of history and suggested that prick or scratch skin testing with food extracts could also help in the identification of food offenders.* They further suggested that blinded physician-supervised oral food challenges were presently "the only unequivocal way of documenting a specific food allergy." However, they noted,

"In some instances where such challenges are not possible, *an elimination diet carried out at home may lead to a clinical diagnosis of food allergy.*"

---

*While prick or scratch tests help identify obvious food allergies, *most individuals with hidden food allergies and other adverse reactions show negative allergy tests to the foods causing their symptoms.*

Hidden Food Allergies and the Yeast Connection

In the fall of 1977, a board certified specialist in internal medicine, C. Orian Truss, M.D. of Birmingham, Alabama told of the relationship of the common yeast, *Candida albicans*, to many chronic health disorders. Symptoms which Dr. Truss found were yeast related ranged from fatigue, headache, depression and premenstrual tension to hyperactivity, inflammatory bowel disease and multiple sclerosis.

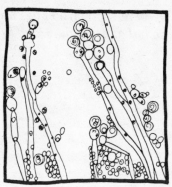

Dr. Truss also reported that a sugar-free, yeast-free special diet and the antifungal medication, nystatin, helped many of his chronically sick patients get well. He published his clinical and research findings in a series of articles in the JOURNAL OF ORTHOMOLECULAR PSYCHIATRY (1978, 1980, 1981, 1984) and in a book, THE MISSING DIAGNOSIS (1983).

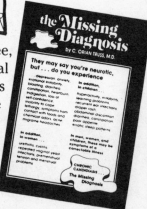

I learned of Dr. Truss' reports in 1979 and began to use his program in my practice. In most of the patients I treated—especially those with fatigue, headache, endocrine dysfunction and a feeling of being "sick all over," I noted a gratifying and often dramatic response. Moreover, hundreds of other physicians and their patients have experienced similar results.

During the past nine years, I have found that many of my patients who are troubled by adverse food reactions give a history of:

1. Repeated or prolonged use of antibiotic drugs and/or corticosteroids.
2. Unusual sensitivity to tobacco smoke, perfumes and other environmental chemicals.

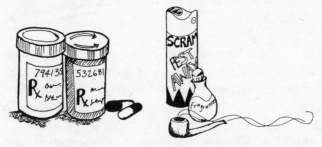

3. Unusual sensitivity to environmental molds.
4. Endocrine problems, especially gonadal and thyroid dysfunction. However, pancreatic dysfunction may also be present as suggested by abnormal fluctuations in blood sugar level and sugar craving.

The Truss observations have now been confirmed by several thousand physicians and other professionals and by countless people with chronic health problems all over the world. Yet, because "appropriate controlled trials which have been approved for scientific merit and safety by competent institutional review boards" haven't yet been carried out, the Practice Standards Committee of the American Academy of Allergy and Immunology has stated,

"The candida-human illness hypothesis is speculative and unproven. The basic elements of the syndrome would apply to almost all sick patients at some time. The complaints are essentially universal; the broad treatment program would produce remission in most illnesses regardless of cause. There is no published proof that *Candida albicans* is responsible for the syndrome."

In spite of this negative evaluation of the yeast-human interaction, there is increasing support for the Truss hypothesis.

In his Foreword to the third edition of THE YEAST CONNECTION, James H. Brodsky, M.D., Chevy Chase, Maryland (Diplomate, American Board of Internal Medicine; Instructor, Georgetown University School of Medicine; American College of Physicians; American Society of Internal Medicine) stated.

"It is time for all physicians and medical scientists to increase their understanding of the relations between yeast and human illness. Many patients with yeast-related health disorders are being treated ineffectively just because their problem has gone unrecognized. *If one reviews the literature carefully, the supporting research is well documented.*"

Brodsky cites twelve articles from the refereed medical literature to document his statements.

Yeast-related changes in mood and behavior have been described by Kazuo Iwata of the University of Tokyo. Along with co-workers, Iwata isolated a potent lethal toxin, *canditoxin,* from a virulent strain of *Candida albicans*.

In his published reports, Iwata found that intravenous injection of the toxin (in mice) caused multiple systemic symptoms including behavioral abnormalities, congestion of eyes, ears and other parts of the body and paralysis of the extremities. He also noted the possibility that "the toxin produced in the invaded tissues may act as an immunosuppressant to impair host defense mechanisms involving cellular immunity."

Dr. E. W. Rosenberg, Professor and Chairman, Division of Dermatology, University of Tennessee Center for the Health Sciences in Memphis, in a brief report in the NEW ENGLAND JOURNAL OF MEDICINE commented,

The New England Journal of Medicine

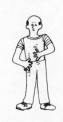

"We've become aware . . . of improvement of both psoriasis and inflammatory bowel disease in patients treated with oral nystatin, an agent that was expected to work only on yeast in the gut lumen. We've now confirmed that observation in several of our patients with psoriasis. *We suspect, therefore, that gut yeast may have a role in some instances of psoriasis."*

Subsequently, Rosenberg and associates and Sidney M. Baker of New Haven, Connecticut, published a report on the successful use of oral nystatin in the treatment of psoriasis. They described the favorable . . . even dramatic . . . response of four patients who had suffered from psoriasis for from ten to forty years.

In 1984, in a 27-page report, C. Orian Truss reported on metabolic abnormalities in 24 of his patients with yeast-related problems. He found that levels of amino acids and fatty acids were abnormal compared to similar studies in asymptomatic patients.

In the May/June, 1985 issue of INFECTIONS IN MEDICINE, Steven S. Witkin published his observations on 50 women who had experienced at least three episodes of candida vaginal infection within a 12-month period. In an article entitled, *Defective Immune Responses in Patients with Recurrent Candidiasis,* Witkin stated,

"Candida albicans infection, often associated with antibiotic-induced alterations in microbial flora, may cause defects in cellular immunity . . . Recent studies suggest that the infection itself may cause immunosuppression resulting in recurrences in certain patients. In addition to creating an increased susceptibility to the candida reinfection, *the immunological alterations may also be*

related to subsequent endocrinopathies and autoantibody formation . . .

"Reports that immunological endocrine abnormalities have been reversed following successful antifungal therapy for candida reinfection lend credence to the idea that these abnormalities can arise as secondary consequences of fungal infection."

Here's a more recent report: Jay S. Schinfeld, Associate Professor, Department of Obstetrics and Gynecology, Temple University School of Medicine, studied thirty-two women with severe premenstrual syndrome (PMS) and a history of vaginal candidiasis. In each patient, prior therapy had failed to help. All patients were treated with an oral anticandidal agent (nystatin) and a yeast elimination diet.

APRIL

H: Headache   B: Bloating
F: Fatigue   I: Irritability
D: Depression

1	2	3	4	5	6	7
8	9	10	11	12	13	14
15	16	17	18	19	20	21
H,F	H,F	H,I,D,F	H,I,D, B,F	H,I, D,F	B,I	B,I
22	23	24	25	26	27	28
START PERIOD						
29	30	31				

"All the patients in the study were long-time PMS sufferers who were felt to have severe symptoms dominated and frequently accompanied by anxiety or anger. Headaches, described as menstrual migraines, were common, as were food cravings, bloating, and significant decreases in libido . . . Treated patients showed significant physical and psychological improvement over untreated controls."

The authors, however, stated that "The mechanism for this improvement and the role of yeast in this disorder remain controversial."

Although the support for the candida-human interaction first described by Truss may not convince skeptics who demand "appropriate controlled trials . . . approved by scientific merit . . . by institutional review boards," it is appropriate to stress the importance of the experience gained by physicians in treating their patients.

Although he did not refer to candida-related disorders, Gene Stollerman, M.D. (Professor of Medicine, Boston University) recently stressed the importance of the observations of the practicing physician. In an editorial in HOSPITAL PRACTICE, he said,

"As the insights of medical bioscience and technology increase our medical powers, I find renewed strength in my clinical skills."

Clinical skills means talking to patients, listening to patients, looking at them and examining them." Dr. Stollerman especially emphasized the medical history which he said would provide more relevant information "as we learn better questions to ask."

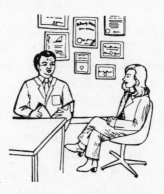

He concluded his comments with this statement, *"Clinical experience is the gold standard on which patient care should be based."*

Along with many other physicians, I am "clinically experienced" in treating and helping many chronically-ill patients using a comprehensive treatment program which includes antifungal therapy and appropriate modification of the diet.

Although new scientific studies may help confirm the role of candida—and of adverse food reactions in making people sick, we should not wait for such studies. Instead, we can learn "better questions to ask" our patients and continue to use our clinical experience and judgement in caring for them. In this way we can help relieve the suffering of many sick people.

Here's more support for clinical observation. In a 1984 article in the JOURNAL OF THE AMERICAN MEDICAL ASSOCIATION, two University of New Mexico physicians published an article which I found fascinating. It's title: *The Tomato Effect* (Goodwin, J. S. and Goodwin, J.M., JAMA 251:2287-2290, May 11, 1984).

According to these two medical school professors, the tomato effect in medicine occurs when an efficacious treatment for a certain disease is ignored or rejected because it does not "make sense." In the article they reviewed a number of examples of the tomato effect in medicine. In their continuing discussion, they commented,

"Modern medicine is particularly vulnerable to the tomato effect. Pharmaceutical companies have . . . turned to theoretical over practical arguments for using their drugs . . . (yet) the only three issues that matter in picking a therapy: *Does it help? How toxic is it? How much does it cost?* In this atmosphere, we're at risk for rejecting a safe, inexpensive, effective therapy in favor of an alternative treatment, perhaps less efficacious and more toxic."

Now then. Back to the relationship of hidden food allergies to health disorders related to *Candida albicans*. To learn more about this relationship I sent a questionnaire to physicians interested in these disorders. Here are two of the questions I asked:

1. Do you often see adverse food reactions in your patients with candida-related health disorders?
2. What foods have you found to be the most common troublemakers?

Twenty-five physicians responded to the questionnaire. *Each respondent noted all of their patients with a candida-related health problem showed an adverse reaction to one or more foods.*

Common troublemakers included yeast, milk, wheat, corn and, to a lesser degree, legumes, eggs, citrus and chocolate.

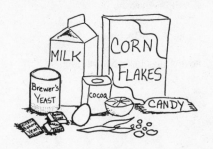

Why would all of these patients with candida-related health problems be troubled with food hypersensitivities? (I'll cite some scientific studies along with my own speculations which I feel may provide us with some answers.)

In the Preface of a 1985 book, *Candidiasis* (edited by Gerald P. Bodey, M.D. and Victor Fainstein, Infectious Disease Section, Department of Internal Medicine, University of Texas) appeared the following statements:

"*Candida spp* have emerged as important pathogens during the past few decades... With the advent of broad spectrum antibiotic therapy, there has been a substantial increase in the number of patients with thrush and vaginitis. These antibiotics alter the normal flora of the body, facilitating colonization and subsequent superinfection by *Candida spp.*"

As previously noted, research studies by both Iwata and Witkin showed that *Candida albicans* infections often associated with antibiotic-induced alterations and microbial flora may cause immunosuppression. So it would seem to me that it would be reasonable to conclude that when the immune system is depressed, food and other hypersensitivities would be more apt to develop.

Here's more. For a number of years, W. Allen Walker, Professor of Pediatrics, Harvard Medical School, has been conducting research on the role of the mucosal barrier in the handling of antigens (allergens) by the gut. His studies indicate that this mucosal barrier can be adversely affected through many different mecha-

O – Normal Gut Flora

Y – Candida Albicans

● – Pathogenic Bacteria

T – Toxins and/or Food antigens

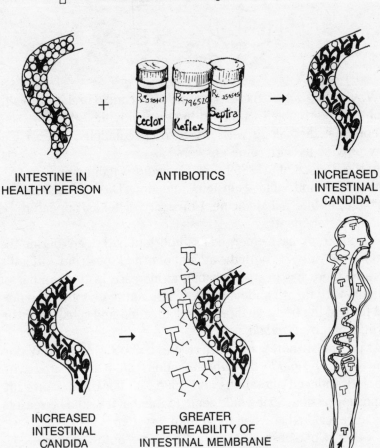

INTESTINE IN
HEALTHY PERSON

+

ANTIBIOTICS

→

INCREASED
INTESTINAL
CANDIDA

INCREASED
INTESTINAL
CANDIDA

→

GREATER
PERMEABILITY OF
INTESTINAL MEMBRANE

→

INCREASED
ABSORPTION
OF TOXINS
AND/OR FOOD
ALLERGENS

nisms. In a recent comprehensive review of antigen handling by the gut, Walker commented,

". . . There is increasing experimental and clinical evidence to suggest that large antigenically-active molecules can penetrate the intestinal epithelial surface, not in sufficient quantities to be of nutritional importance, but in quantities that may be of immunological importance.

"This observation could mean that the intestinal tract represents a potential site for the absorption of bacterial breakdown products such as endotoxins and enterotoxins, of proteolytic and hydrolytic enzymes or other ingested food antigens that normally exist in the intestinal lumen . . ."

Walker does not mention the possible role of candida in compromising the mucosal barrier leading to the increased absorption of ingested food antigens. Yet, the observations of Bodey, Fainstein, Iwata and Witkin suggest—to me—that excessive candida colonization and/or infection in the gut could lead to the absorption of more food allergens.

Moreover, I have found that many of my food-sensitive patients regain tolerance to their food troublemakers following a comprehensive antifungal treatment program. Such a program features a nutritious, rotated, diversified, sugar-free diet, antifungal therapy with nystatin (and/or Nizoral) and appropriate lifestyle changes.

Reading List

On Allergy, Immunology, Environmental Medicine and Nutrition. Contemporary Books of Interest to Professional and Non-Professionals.

*Bahna, S. L. and Heiner, D. C.: *Allergies to Milk,* Springfield, Illinois, Charles C. Thomas, 1980.

*Breneman, J. C.: Handbook of Food Allergies, New York, Marcel Dekker, Inc. 1987

Brody, Jane: *Jane Brody's Good Food Book,* New York, Bantam Books edition, 1987.

*Brostoff, J. and Challacombe, S. J.: *Food Allergy and Intolerance,* Ballière Tindall, 33 D Avenue, Eastbourne, East Sussex, BN21 3UN England.

Callahan, Mary: *Fighting for Tony,* Simon and Schuster, New York, Fireside Books, 1987.

Crook, W. G.: *Are You Allergic?* (former title: *Your Allergic Child*), Jackson, Tennessee, Professional Books, 1978 (revised).

Crook, W. G. and Stevens, L.: *Solving the Puzzle of Your Hard-to-Raise Child,* New York, Random House and Jackson, Tennessee, Professional Books, 1987.

Crook, W. G.: *The Yeast Connection,* New York, Vintage Books and Jackson, Tennessee, Professional Books, Third Edition, Paperback, 1986.

Davies, S. and Stewart, A.: *Nutritional Medicine,* London, Pan Books, 1987.

Faelten, S. and editors of Prevention Magazine: *Allergy Self-Help Book,* Emmaus, Pennsylvania, Rodale Press, 1983.

Feingold, B. F.: *Why Your Child is Hyperactive,* New York, Random House, 1974.

Forman, R.: *How to Control Your Allergies,* New York, New York, Larchmont Book Company, 1979.

Frazier, C. A.: *Coping with Food Allergy, Revised edition* New York, The New York Times Book Company, 1985.

Galland, L.: *Superimmunity for Kids,* New York, Dutton, 1988.

Gerrard, J. W. (ed.): *Understanding Allergies*, Springfield, Illinois, Charles C. Thomas, 1973.

*Gerrard, J. W. (ed.): *Food Allergy: New Perspectives*, Springfield, Illinois, Charles C. Thomas, 1980.

Goldbeck, N. and D.: *The Goldbeck's Guide To Good Food*, New York, New American Library, 1987.

Golos, N. and Golbitz, F. G.: *Coping with Your Allergies* (Revised paperback edition), New York, Simon and Schuster, 1985.

Golos, N. and Golbitz, F. G.: *If This is Tuesday, It Must Be Chicken*, 1981. Available from Human Ecology Research Foundation of the Southwest, 12110 Webbs Chapel Road, Suite 305, East, Dallas, Texas 75234.

*Hare, F.: *The Food Factor in Disease*, London, Longmans, Green and Company, Volumes I and II, 1905.

Hill, A. N.: *Against the Unsuspected Enemy*, London, New Horizon, 1980.

Hunter, B. T.: *Additive Books*, New Canaan, Connecticut, Keats Publishing, 1980.

Jones, M. H.: *The Allergy Self-Help Cookbook*, Emmaus, Pennsylvania, Rodale Press, 1984.

Kane, P.: *Food Makes the Difference*, New York, Simon and Schuster, 1985.

Levin, A. S. and Zellerback, M.: *Type 1/Type 2 Allergy Relief Program*, Los Angeles, California, Jeremy D. Tarcher, Inc., Distributed by Houghton Mifflin Company, Boston, Massachusetts, 1983.

Mackarness, R.: *Eating Dangerously: The Hazards of Hidden Allergies*, New York, Harcourt, Brace, Jovanovich, 1976.

Mackarness, R.: *Not All In The Mind*, London, Pan Books, 1976.

Mandell, M. and Scanlon, L.: *Dr. Mandell's 5-Day Allergy Relief System*, New York, Pocket Books, 1979.

Mandell, M.: *Dr. Mandell's Lifetime Arthritis Relief System*, New York, Coward-McCann, 1983.

Mansfield, J.: *The Migraine Revolution*, Wellingborough and New York, Thorson Publishing Group, 1986.

McGee, C. T.: *How to Survive Modern Technology*, Alamo, California, Ecology Press, p. 11, 1979.

Mumby, K.: *The Food Allergy Plan*, London, Unwin, 1985.

Oski, F.: *Don't Drink Your Milk*, New York, Wyden Books. 1977 and Syracuse, New York, Molica Press. 1983.

Philpott, W. H. and Kalita, B. K.: *Brain Allergies*, New Canaan, Connecticut, Keats Publishing, 1980.

Price, W. A.: *Nutrition and Physical Degeneration*, Berkeley, CA, Parker House, 1981. (Available from Price-Pottenger Foundation, Post Office Box 2614, La Mesa, CA 92014.)

Randolph, T. G. and Moss, R.: *An Alternative Approach to Allergies*, New York, Harper and Row, 1980.

Rapp, D. J.: *Allergies and The Hyperactive Child*, New York, Cornerstone, 1980.

Rapp, D. J.: *Allergies and Your Family*, New York, Sterling Publishing Company, 1981.

Rapp, D. J.: *The Impossible Child*, Tacoma, Washington, Life Sciences Press, 1986. (Available from Practical Allergy Research Foundation, Post Office Box 60, Buffalo, New York 14223.)

Rippere, V.: *The Allergy Problem, Why People Suffer and What Should Be Done*, Wellingborough, Northhamptonshire, England, Thorson Publishers, Ltd., 1983.

Rogers, S. A.: *The EI Syndrome*, Prestige Publishers, Box 3161, Syracuse, New York, 1986.

Sheinkin, D., Schacter, and Hutton, R.: *Food Mind and Mood*, New York, Warner Books, 1980.

Sloan, S.: *The Brown Bag Cookbook*, Charlotte, Vermont, Williamson Publishing, 1984.

*Speer, F.: *Food Allergy*, Littleton, Massachusetts, PSG Publishing Company, 1983 (Second Edition).

*Speer, F.: *Allergy of the Nervous System*, Springfield, Illinois, Charles C. Thomas, 1970.

Stevens, L. J.: *The Complete Book of Allergy Control*, New York, New York, MacMillan Publishing Company, 1983.

Williams, R. J.: *Physicians Handbook of Nutritional Science*, Springfield, Illinois, Charles C. Thomas, 1978.

Wunderlich, R. and Kalita, D.: *Nourishing Your Child*, New Canaan, Connecticut, Keats Publishing, 1984.

Wunderlich, R. C., Jr.: *Sugar and Your Health*, Johnny Reads, Inc., St. Petersburg, Florida, Good Health Publications, 1982.

---

*Denotes books of special interest to physicians.

References

Alvarez, W. C.: In Speer, F.: *Allergies of the Nervous System,* Springfield, Illinois, Charles C. Thomas, 1970, pp. ix-xi.

Alvarez, W. C.: "Puzzling 'Nervous Storms' Due to Food Allergy," *Gastro-Enterology,* 7:241, 1946.

"American Academy of Allergy and Immunology, Position Statement, Candidiasis Hypersensitivity Syndrome," *J. of Allergy and Clinical Immunology,* 78:271, August, 1986.

Bahna, S. L. and Heiner, D. C.: *Allergies to Milk,* Springfield, Illinois, Charles C. Thomas, 1980, pp. 67-71.

Bodey, G. P. and Fainstein, D.: *Candidiasis,* New York, Raven Press, 1985.

Bray, G. W.: "Enuresis of Allergic Origin," *Arch. Dis. Child.,* 1931, 6:251, 1951.

Breneman, J. C.: "Allergic Cystitis: The Cause of Nocturnal Enuresis," *G.P.,* 20:84, 1959.

Breneman, J. C.: "Nocturnal Enuresis: A Treatment Regimen For General Use," *Annals of Allergy,* 23:185-191, 1965.

Breneman, J. C.: *Basics of Food Allergy,* Springfield, Illinois, Charles C. Thomas, Second Edition, 1984.

Brodsky, J. N.: In Crook, W. G.: *The Yeast Connection* (Foreword), Third Edition, Jackson, Tennessee, Professional Books and New York, Random House, 1986.

Brostoff, J. and Challacombe, S. J.: *Food Allergy and Intolerance,* London, Ballière Tindall, and Pennsylvania, W. B. Saunders, 1987.

Bullock, J. D., Deamer, W. C., Frick, O. L., Crisp, J. R., III, Galant, S. P., and Ziering, W. H.: "Recurrent Abdominal Pain" (letters), *Pediatrics,* 46:969, 1970.

Campbell, M. B.: "Neurologic Manifestations of Allergic Disease," *Annals of Allergy,* 31:485, 1973.

Clarke, T. W.: "The Relationship of Allergy to Character Problems in Children: A Survey," *Ann. Allergy,* 8:175, 1950.

Clein, N. W.: "Cow's Milk Allergy in Infants," *Pediatric Clinics in Amer.,* 1:949, 1954.

Coca, A. F.: *Familial Non-Reaginic Food Allergy,* Springfield, Illinois, Charles C. Thomas, 1942.

Crook, W. G., Harrison, W. W., Crawford, S. E., and Emerson, B. S.: "Systemic Manifestations Due to Allergy. Report of Fifty Patients and a Review of the Literature on the Subject," *Pediatrics*, 27:790–799, 1961.

Crook, W. G.: "The Allergic Tension-Fatigue Syndrome." In Speer, F. (ed.): *The Allergic Child*, New York, Hoeber, 1963.

Crook, W. G.: "Recurrent Abdominal Pain" (letters), *Pediatrics*, 46:969, 1970.

Crook, W. G.: "Adverse Reactions to Food Can Cause Hyperkinesis" (letters), *American Journal of Dis. Child.*, 132:819, 1978.

Crook, W. G.: "School Phobia? Or Allergic Tension-Fatigue?" (letters), *Pediatrics*, 50:340, 1972.

Crook, W. G.: "Musculoskeletal Allergy, Genitourinary Allergy." In Speer, F. and Dockhorn, R. (ed.): *Allergy and Immunology in Children*, Springfield, Illinois, Charles C. Thomas, 1973.

Crook, W. G.: "The Allergic Tension-Fatigue Syndrome," *Pediatric Annals*, October, 1974.

Crook, W. G.: *Are You Allergic?: A Guide to Normal Living for Allergic Adults and Children*, Jackson, Tennessee, Professional Books, 1975.

Crook, W. G.: "Food Allergy—the Great Masquerader," *Pediatric Clinics of North America*, 22:227, 1975.

Crook, W. G.: "Many Pediatricians See a Relationship Between Diet, Hyperactivity," *Pediatric News*, 13:1, July, 1979.

Crook, W. G.: "Hidden Food Allergy, A Common and Often Unrecognized Cause of Chronic Symptoms in Children," Scientific Exhibit, American Academy of Pediatrics, Annual Meeting, San Francisco, October 14–17, 1979.

Crook, W. G.: "What is Scientific Proof?," *Pediatrics*, 65:638, 1980.

Crook, W. G.: "Can What a Child Eats Make Him Dull, Stupid or Hyperactive?," *Journal of Learning Disabilities*, 13:281, 1980.

Crook, W. G.: "Hidden Food Allergy, A Common and Often Unrecognized Cause of Chronic Symptoms in Children," Scientific Exhibit, American Academy of Pediatrics, Annual Meeting, New Orleans, October, 1981.

Crook, W. G.: "Diet and Hyperactivity," *Clinical Pediatrics* (letters), 68:300, 1981.

Crook, W. G.: "Childhood Depression and Diet," *Amer. J. Dis. Children*, 136:652, 1982.

Crook, W. G.: "The Coming Revolution in Medicine," *Tennessee Medical Association*, 73:3, March, 1983.

Daniel 1:1–20, *Good News Bible: The Bible in Today's English Version*, New York, New York, American Bible Society, 1976, pp. 954–955.

Davison, H. M.: "Allergy of the Nervous System," *Quarterly Review Allergy*, 6:157, 1952.

Davison, H. M.: "Cerebral Allergy," *Southern Med. J.*, 42:712, 1947.

Deamer, W. C.: "Recurrent Abdominal Pain," *Current Medical Digest,* February, 1973.

Deamer, W. C.: "Pediatric Allergy: Some Impressions Gained over a 37-Year Period," *Pediatrics,* 48:930, 1971.

Deamer, W. C.: "Recurrent Abdominal Pain: Recurrent Controversy" (letters), *Pediatrics* 46:307, 1973.

Dees, S. C.: "Neurologic Allergy in Childhood," *Pediatric Clinics of North America,* 1:1017, 1954.

Dees, S. and Lowenbach, H.: "The Electroencephalograms of Allergic Children," *Annals of Allergy,* 6:99, 1948.

Duke, W. W.: "Food Allergy as a Cause of Illness," *JAMA,* 81:886, 1923.

Duke, W. W.: *Allergy, Asthma, Hayfever, Urticaria and other Allied Manifestations of Reaction,* St. Louis, Mosby, 1925.

Egger, J., Carter, C. M., Wilson, J., Soothill, J., et al: "Is Migraine Food Allergy? A Double-Blind Trial of Oligoantigenic Diet Treatment," *Lancet,* 1983, ii:865.

Egger, J., Carter, C. M., Graham, P. J., et al: "Controlled Trial of Oligoantigenic Diet Treatment in the Hyperkinetic Syndrome," *Lancet,* 1985, i:540–5.

Galland, L.: *Superimmunity for Kids,* New York, Dutton, 1988.

Gerrard, J. W.: *Understanding Allergies,* Springfield, Illinois, Charles C. Thomas, 1973.

Gerrard, J. W.: "Nocturnal Enuresis." In Gerrard, J. W. (ed.): *Food Allergy: New Perspectives,* Springfield, Illinois, Charles C. Thomas, 1980.

Gerrard, J. W., Heiner, D. C., Ives, E. J., and Hardy, L. W.: "Milk Allergy: Recognition, Natural History and Management," *Clinical Pediatrics,* 2:634, 1963.

Gerrard, J. W. and Esperance, M.: "Nocturnal Enuresis: Studies in Bladder Function in Normals and Enuretics," *Canadian Medical Association Journal,* 101:269, 1969.

Grant, E. E. C.: "Food Allergies and Migraine," *Lancet,* 1979, i:966–9.

Hare, F.: *The Food Factor in Disease,* London, Longmans, Green and Company, 1905.

Hedges, H.: *Jour. Ark. Med. Soc.,* 78:930–938, 1971.

Hill, D.: "Food Allergy and Arthritis," Presentation, American College of Allergists, Conference on Food Allergy, Atlanta 1984.

Hilsen, J. M.: "Dietary Control of the Hyperactive Child," *Long Island Pediatrician* (Summer, 1982), pp. 25–32.

Hippocrates. As quoted by Bell, I. R.: *Clinical Ecology,* Bolinas, CA, Common Knowledge Press, 1982, p. 7.

Hoobler, B. R.: "Some Early Symptoms Suggesting Protein Sensitization in Infancy," *American J. of Dis. of Child.,* 12:129, 1916.

Iwata, K. and Yamamoto, Y.: "Glycoprotein Toxins Produced by Candida Albi-

cans," Proceedings of the Fourth International Conference on the My-
coses, June, 1977, *PAHO Scientific Publication #356.*

Iwata, K.: *In Recent Advances in Medical and Veterinary Mycology,* University
of Tokyo Press, 1977.

Iwata, K. and Uchida, K.: "Cellular Immunity in Experimental Fungus Infections in Mice," *Medical Mycology Flims,* January, 1977.

Jones, V. A. and Hunter, J. O.: "Irritable Bowel Syndrome and Crohn's Disease." In Brostoff J. and Challacombe S. J,: *Food Allergy and Intolerance,*
London, Ballière Tindall, Philadelphia, London and W. B. Saunders,
1987, pp. 555–569.

Kemp, J. P.: "Recurrent Abdominal Pain" (letters), *Pediatrics,* 46:969, 1970.

Kniker, W. T.: "Deciding the Future for the Practice of Allergy and Immunology," *Annals of Allergy,* 55:106–113, 1985.

Kniker, W. T.: "Food Allergy," Presentation at Annual Meeting of the American
College of Allergists, Phoenix, Arizona, January, 1986.

Kniker, W. T.: "Food Allergy" (workshop), 44th Annual Meeting, American
College of Allergists, Boston, November, 1987.

Kroker, G., Stroud, R. M., and Marshall, R., et al: "Fasting and Rheumatoid
Arthritis: A Multi-Center Study," *Arch. of Clin. Ecology,* Volume 2, Number 3, pp. 137–144, 1984.

Kroker, G. F.: "Chronic Candidiasis and Allergy." In Brostoff, J. and Challacombe, S. J.: *Food Allergy and Intolerance,* Philadelphia, Ballière Tindall
and London, W. B. Saunders, 1987.

Marshall, R., Stroud, R. M., and Kroker, G.: "Food Challenge Effects on Fasted
Rheumatoid Arthritis Patients: A Multi-Center Study," Volume 2,
Number 4, pp. 181–190, 1984. Also presented at the third annual sympo-
sium on food allergy, American College of Allergists, Boston, 1982.

Matsumura, T., et al: "Significance of Food Allergy in the Etiology of Orthos-
tatic Albuminuria," *Journal of Asthma Research,* 3:325, 1966.

Matsumura, T. and Kuromi, T.: "The Role of Allergy in the Pathogenesis of the
Nephrotic Syndrome," *J. Pediatr.,* 14:921, 1961.

Marks, M. B.: "Nasal Allergy in Childhood: The Observations in the South
Florida Area," *Ann. Allergy,* 18:1110, 1960.

Marks, M. B.: "The Gaping Allergic Child," *Ann. Allergy,* 23:616, 1965.

Marks, M. B.: "Allergic Shiners: Dark Circles Under the Eyes in Children,"
Clin. Pediatr., 5:655, 1966.

Marks, M. B.: (Introduction), *Stigmata of Respiratory Tract Allergies,* edited by
Thomas, B. A., published by the Upjohn Company, Kalamazoo, Michigan,
1967, 1972 and 1977.

May, E.: "Attacks of Unnatural Somnolence of Anaphylactic Origin," *Bull. Soc.
Med. Hop.,* Paris, 47:704, 1923.

McGovern, J. P. and Haywood, T. J.: "Allergic Headache." In Speer, F.: *Allergy and the Nervous System,* Springfield, Illinois, Charles C. Thomas, 1970, pp. 47–58.

Menzies, I. C.: "Disturbed Children: The Role of Food in Chemical Sensitivities," *Nutr. In Health,* 3:39–54, 1984, Academic Publishers. Printed in Great Britain.

Monro, J., Carini, C., and Brostoff, J.: "Migraine is a Food Allergic Disease," *Lancet,* 1984, ii:719–721.

Monro, J.: "Food Induced Migraine." In Brostoff, J. and Challacombe, S. J.: *Food Allergy and Intolerance,* London, Ballière Tindall, 1987, p. 633–665.

Monro, J. and others: "Food Allergy in Migraine," *Lancet,* Volume 8184, July 5, 1980, pp. 104.

O'Banion, B. R.: "Dietary Control of Headache Pain: Five Case Studies," *J. Holistic Medicine,* 3:140–151, 1982.

O'Banion, B. R.: "Dietary Control of Rheumatoid Arthritis Pain: Three Case Studies," *J. Holistic Medicine,* 4:49–57, 1982.

Ogle, K. and Bullock, J. D.: "Children with Allergic Rhinitis and/or Bronchial Asthma Treated with Elimination Diet: A Five-Year Follow Up," *Annals of Allergy,* 44:273, 1980.

Oski, F. and Bell, J. D.: *Don't Drink Your Milk,* Wyden Books, 1977, pp. 63–65.

Oster, J.: "Recurrent Abdominal Pain, Headache, and Limb Pains in Children and Adolescents," *Pediatrics,* 50:429, 1972.

Panush, R., Stroud, R. M., and Webster, E. M.: "Food Induced (Allergic) Arthritis, Inflammatory Arthritis Exacerbated by Milk," *Arthritis Rheum.,* 29:220–6, 1986.

Piness, G. and Miller, H.: "Allergic Manifestations in Infancy and Childhood," *Arch. Pediat.,* 42:557, 1925.

Poley, J. R. and Bhatia M.: *Pediatrics,* 52:142, 1973.

Pounders, C. M.: "The Life Cycle of the Allergic Individuals," *Southern Med. J.,* 45:875, 1952.

Prinz, R. J., Roberts, W. A., and Hantman, E.: "Dietary Correlates of Hyperactive Behavior in Children," *Journal of Consulting Clinical Psychologists,* 48:769, 1980.

Randolph, T. G.: "Allergies as a Causative Factor of Fatigue, Irritability, and Behavior Problems in Children," *Journal of Pediatrics,* 32:266, 1948.

Randolph, T. G.: "Fatigue and Weakness of Allergic Origin (Allergic Toxemia) to be Differentiated from Nervous Fatigue and Neurasthenia," *Annals of Allergy,* 3:418, 1945.

Randolph, T. G. and Moss, R.: *An Alternative Approach to Allergies,* New York, Bantam, 1982, p. 50.

Rapp, D. J.: "Does Diet Affect Hyperactivity?" *Journal of Learning Disabilities,* 11:56–61, 1978.

Rapp, D. J.: *Allergies and the Hyperactive Child,* New York, New York, Sovereign Books, 1979.

Rapp, D. J. and Bamberg, D.: *The Impossible Child,*Practical Allergy Research Foundation, Buffalo, New York 1986.

Rapp, D. J.: "Food Allergy and Hyperactivity." In Gerrard, J. W. (ed.): *Food Allergy: New Perspectives,* Springfield, Illinois, Charles C. Thomas, 1980.

Rapp, D. J.: "Elimination Diets and Hyperactivity," *Pediatrics,* 67:937, 1981 (letters).

Rinkel, H. J., Randolph, T., and Zeller, M.: *Food Allergy: New Perspectives,* Springfield, Illinois, Charles C. Thomas, 1951. (Republished by the New England Foundation for Allergic and Environmental Diseases, Norwalk, Connecticut, 1980.)

Rinkel, H. J.: "Food Allergy: The Role of Food Allergy in Internal Medicine," *Annals of Allergy,* 2:115, 1944.

Rinkel, H. J.: "Food Allergy, The Technique and Clinical Application of Individual Food Tests," *Annals of Allergy,* 2:504, 1944.

Rinkel, H. J.: "The Function and Clinical Application of the Rotary Diversified Diet," *J. Ped.,* 32:266, 1948.

Rinkel, H. J., Randolph, T. G., and Zeller, M.: *Food Allergy,* Springfield, Illinois, Charles C. Thomas, 1951.

Rinkel, H. J.: "The Diagnosis of Food Allergy," *Archives of Otolaryngology,* Volume 79, 1964, p. 71.

Rosenberg, E. W. (and associates): (Letters) "Crohn's Disease and Psoriasis," *New England Journal of Medicine,* Volume 308(2), 61–112, January 13, 1983.

Rosenberg, E. W., et al and Baker, S.: *Archives of Dermatology,* 1984.

Rowe, A. H., Sr.: "Allergic Toxemia and Migraine Due to Food Allergy," *California Western Medicine,* Volume 33, 1930, p. 785.

Rowe, A. H., Sr.: *Food Allergy: Its Manifestations, Diagnosis and Treatment,* Philadelphia, Lea and Febiger, 1931.

Rowe, A. H., Sr.: "Chronic Ulcerative Colitis, Allergy in its Etiology," *Annals of Internal Medicine,* 17:83, 1942.

Rowe, A. H.: *Elimination Diets and the Patient's Allergies,* Philadelphia, Lee and Febiger, 1944.

Rowe, A. H.: "Clinical Allergy and the Nervous System," *J. Neru. Ment. Dis.,* 99:834, 1944.

Rowe, A. H.: "Allergic Toxemia and Fatigue,." *Annals of Allergy,* 8:72, 1950.

Rowe, A. H.: "Allergic Toxemia and Fatigue," *Annals of Allergy,* 17:9, 1959.

Rowe, A. H. and Rowe, A. H., Jr.: "Perennial Nasal Allergy Due to Food Sensitivity," *J. of Asth. Research,* 3:141, 1965.

Rowe, A. H., Rowe, A., Jr.: *Food Allergy: It's Manifestations and Control and the Elimination Diets.* A Compendium. Springfield, Illinois, Charles C. Thomas, 1972.

Sandberg, D. H.: "Recurrent Abdominal Pain: Recurrent Controversy" (letters), *Pediatrics,* 51:307, 1973.

Sampson, H. A., Buckley, R. H., and Metcalf, D. D.: "Food Allergy," *JAMA,* 258:2886–2890, 1987.

Sandberg, D. H.: "Recurrent Abdominal Pain, Recurrent Controversy," *Pediatrics,* 51:307, 1973.

Sandberg, D. H.: "Food Sensitivity: The Kidney and Bladder." In Brostoff, J. and Challacombe, S. J.: Food and Intolerance, London, Ballière Tindall, pp. 755–767.

Sandberg, D. H., McLeod, P. F., and Strauss, J.: "Renal Disease Related to Hypersensitivity to Foods." In Gerrard, J. W. (ed.): *Food Allergy: New Perspectives,* Springfield, Illinois, Charles C. Thomas, 1980, p. 144.

Schmitt, B.: "School Phobia—The Great Imitator: A Pediatrician's Point of View," *Pediatrics,* 48:433, 1971.

Schinfeld, J. S.: "PMS and Candidiasis: Study Explores Possible Link," *The Female Patient,* 12:66, 1987.

Schoenthaler, S.: "The Effect of Sugar on the Treatment and Control of Antisocial Behavior: A Double-Blind Study of an Incarcerated Juvenile Population," *The International Journal for Biosocial Research,* 3:1, 1982.

Shambaugh, G. E., Jr.: "Serous Otitis: Are Tubes the Answer?", *Amer. J. of Otol.,* 5:63, 1983.

Shambaugh, G. E. Jr.: "History of Allergy in Otolaryngology," Shambaugh Medical Research Institute, 1984. 40 South Clay Street, Hinsdale, Illinois

Shannon, W. R.: "Neuropathic Manifestations in Infants and Children as a Result of Anaphylactic Reactions to Foods Contained in Their Dietary," *American Journal of Diseases of Children,* Volume 24, 1922, p. 89.

Speer, F.: "The Allergic Tension-Fatigue Syndrome," *Pediatric Clinics of North America,* Volume 1, 1954, p. 1029.

Speer, F.: "The Allergic Tension-Fatigue Syndrome in Children," *International Archives of Allergy,* Volume 12, 1958, p. 207.

Speer, F.: *Allergy of the Nervous System,* Springfield, Illinois, Charles C. Thomas, 1980.

Speer, F.: *Food Allergy,* Littleton, Massachusetts, PSG Publishing Company, Second Edition, 1983.

Stollerman, G. H.: "The Gold Standard," *Hospital Practice,* Volume 20, January 30, 1985, p. 9.

Stone, R. T. and Barbero, G. J.: "Recurrent Abdominal Pain in Childhood," *Pediatrics,* 45:732, 1970.

Stroud, R. M.: "The Effects of Fasting Followed by Specific Food Challenge on

Rheumatoid Arthritis in Current Topics and Rheumatology, A Collection of Johns-Hopkins Fellows, Past and Present," Upjohn, 1983, pp. 145–157.

Tolber, S. G.: "Food Problems," *Cutis,* 28:360, 1981.

Truss, C. O.: "Tissue Injury Induced by C. Albicans: Mental and Neurologic Manifestations," *Journal of Orthomolecular Psychiatry,* 7:17–37, 1978.

Truss, C. O.: "Restoration of Immunologic Competence to C. Albicans," *Journal of Orthomolecular Psychiatr,* 9:287–301, 1980.

Truss, C. O.: "The Role of Candida Albicans in Human Illness," *Journal of Orthomolecular Psychiatr,* 10:228–238, 1981.

Truss, C. O.: "Metabolic Abnormalitites in Patients with Chronic Candidiasis," *Journal of Orthomolecular Psychiatr,* 13:66–93, 1984.

Truss, C. O.: *The Missing Diagnosis,* Post Office Box 26508, Birmingham, Alabama 35226, 1983.

Tunnessen, W., Jr.: *Clini-Pearls,* 2:6, August, 1979.

Walker, W. A.: "Role of the Mucosal Barrier in Antigen Handling by the Gut." In Brostoff, J. and Challacombe, S. J.: *Food Allergy and Intolerance,* London, Ballière Tindall, 1987, pp. 209–222.

Witkin, S.: *Infections in Medicine,* May/June 1985, pp. 129-132.

Ordering Information

You'll find Dr. Crook's publications in many bookstores, health food stores and pharmacies.

The Yeast Connection
Expanded and updated third edition, trade paperback	**$ 7.95**
Expanded and updated third edition, hardback	**$13.95**

Booklets
Yeasts . . . and How They Can Make You Sick	**$ 1.95**
Allergy . . . How It Affects You and Your Child	**$ 1.95**
Hypoglycemia . . . (Low Blood Sugar)	**$ 1.95**
Hard-To-Raise Children . . . and How to Help Them	**$ 1.95**

Other Books
Tracking Down Hidden Food Allergy	**$ 6.95**
The Yeast Connection Cookbook (available soon)	
Are You Allergic?	**$ 6.95**
Solving The Puzzle of Your Hard-to-Raise Child	**$17.95**
Detecting Your Hidden Allergies	**$11.95**

ASK ABOUT OUR QUANTITY DISCOUNT PRICES

ORDER FORM

ITEM	QTY.	PRICE	TOTAL
The Yeast Connection			
BOOKLETS: Yeasts			
Allergy			
Hypoglycemia			
Hard-To-Raise Children			
OTHER BOOKS: Tracking Down Hidden Food Allergy			
The Yeast Connection Cookbook		(available	soon)
Are You Allergic?			
Solving The Puzzle of Your Hard-to- Raise Child			
Detecting Your Hidden Allergies			
Add $1.05 for handling of single orders:			
Prices subject to change. **GRAND TOTAL**			

Name   Phone

Street address

City   State   Zip

Send your check or money order with this form to:

Professional Books, P.O. Box 846, Jackson, Tennessee 38302
Tennessee residents add 7% sales tax

Ordering Information

You'll find Dr. Crook's publications in many bookstores, health food stores and pharmacies.

The Yeast Connection
    Expanded and updated third edition, trade paperback   **$ 7.95**
    Expanded and updated third edition, hardback   **$13.95**
Booklets
    Yeasts . . . and How They Can Make You Sick   **$ 1.95**
    Allergy . . . How It Affects You and Your Child   **$ 1.95**
    Hypoglycemia . . . (Low Blood Sugar)   **$ 1.95**
    Hard-To-Raise Children . . . and How to Help Them   **$ 1.95**
Other Books
    Tracking Down Hidden Food Allergy   **$ 6.95**
    The Yeast Connection Cookbook   (available soon)
    Are You Allergic?   **$ 6.95**
    Solving The Puzzle of Your Hard-to-Raise Child   **$17.95**
    Detecting Your Hidden Allergies   **$11.95**

ASK ABOUT OUR QUANTITY DISCOUNT PRICES

ORDER FORM

ITEM	QTY.	PRICE	TOTAL
The Yeast Connection			
BOOKLETS: Yeasts			
Allergy			
Hypoglycemia			
Hard-To-Raise Children			
OTHER BOOKS: Tracking Down Hidden Food Allergy			
The Yeast Connection Cookbook		(available	soon)
Are You Allergic?			
Solving The Puzzle of Your Hard-to- Raise Child			
Detecting Your Hidden Allergies			
Add $1.05 for handling of single orders:			
Prices subject to change.		**GRAND TOTAL**	

Name   Phone

Street address

City   State   Zip

Send your check or money order with this form to:

Professional Books, P.O. Box 846, Jackson, Tennessee 38302
Tennessee residents add 7% sales tax